MRCPCH Part 2
PAEDIATRIC

PRACTICE EXAMS

Dr P Gringras
Consultant Paediatrician
Multiple Births Foundation
Queen Charlotte's Hospital
London
Harper House Children's Service
Hertfordshire

Dr D K Pal
Specialist Registrar in Paediatric Neurology
Great Ormond Street Children's Hospital
London

Dr M Greenberg
Specialist Registrar in Paediatric Gastroenterology
The Royal Free Hospital
London

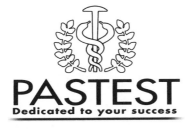

PASTEST
Dedicated to your success

First published 1993
Reprinted 1994, 1995
Second Edition 1999
Reprinted 2000

ISBN 1 901198 26 X

A catalogue record for this book is available from the British Library.

The information contained within this book was obtained by the authors from reliable sources. However, while every effort has been made to ensure its accuracy, no responsibilty for loss, damage or injury occasioned to any person acting or refraining from action as a result of information contained herein can be accepted by the publishers or authors.

PasTest Revision Books and Intensive Courses

PasTest has been established in the field of postgraduate medical education since 1972, providing revision books and intensive study courses for doctors preparing for their professional examinations.

Books and courses are available for the following specialties:

MRCP Part 1 and Part 2, MRCPCH Part 1 and Part 2, MRCOG, DRCOG, MRCGP, DCH, FRCA, MRCS and PLAB.

For further details contact:

PasTest, Freepost, Knutsford, Cheshire WA16 7BR
Tel: 01565 752000   Fax: 01565 650264

Text prepared by Turner Associates, Caistor, Lincoln.
Typeset by Breeze Limited, Manchester.
Printed and bound by Cromwell Press, Trowbridge.

CONTENTS

FOREWORD TO SECOND EDITION

'**Much wisdom I learned from my teachers, more from my colleagues, from my pupils most of all**'.

A career in paediatrics starts with entry to the Specialist Registrar Grade. To achieve this the potential paediatrician must pass the Membership examination of the Royal College of Paediatrics and Child Health, or the Royal College of Physicians.

This book does not guarantee success, but it gives its reader the edge. To acquire the knowledge base required, the candidate must not only be well read, but retain sufficient facts to convince the examiner that they will be a safe and competent practitioner.

Knowledge does not come easily. This book seeks to test the candidate in a meaningful way, by presenting clinical facts in the context of stimulating case histories, testing data which has clinical validity and presenting answers that satisfy even the mature clinicians need to learn. This book has a style that encourages the student to retain facts by making the learning relevant.

As a paediatric teacher and lifelong paediatric learner, this book refines the key competencies required to both pass the dreaded MRCPCH and to be a better informed paediatrician.

Dr A Raffles
Consultant Paediatrician
Queen Elizabeth II Hospital
Hertfordshire

FOREWORD

It is right that those intending to specialize in paediatrics should have their basic knowledge of the subject tested, so that they, as well as their supervisors and employers, can be reassured that their future is likely to be secure.

The examination for the MRCPCH can be a formidable hurdle for newly-qualified doctors who are, sadly, often over-worked and short of sleep. The authors of this book have recently surmounted this hurdle and have set out to help others do so as well.

Clear practical guidance on the written parts of the exam is provided. The book also makes a good (and challenging!) read for those who passed it long ago.

Osmund Reynolds

Professor E.O.R. Reynolds FRS
Professor of Neonatal Paediatrics
University College School of Medicine
London WC1

PREFACE

When this book was first published the authors still had recent and painful memories from taking the MRCP Part 2 Paediatrics examination. As time has passed they have become increasingly more specialised (knowing more and more about less and less) and the prospect of updating the book became more daunting. It was therefore a great delight (and relief) to meet an excellent paediatrician, recently over the MRCP hurdle and keen to contribute to this second edition. Two whole papers contain entirely new material and we have Michael to thank for most of this. We make no apologies for not removing existing questions. They still contain themes that repeatedly recur in the examination and feedback from past successful candidates has been good. We have updated answers as necessary and referenced grey cases. We remain jointly responsible for all the questions in this second edition and would welcome any criticisms that may improve it.

Paul Gringras
Deb Pal
Michael Greenberg

INTRODUCTION : THE WRITTEN EXAMINATION

The overall pass rate for the MRCP (UK) Part 2 (which from September 1999 will become the MRCPCH Part 2) is about 30% with variation between colleges. The written part of the MRCPCH is not a simple hurdle into the 'main' clinical section. It is in fact the written section that provides the most scope for maximising your score.

35% of candidates will fail the written section outright and will not qualify to enter for the clinical examination. However, 15% score a '9' or bare fail in the written section and will be allowed to enter the clinical section. A bare fail in the written section must be balanced by 2 extra marks in the clinical section, a daunting task (no official figures available). A fail in the clinical section cannot be offset by high marks in the written section. Thus it is paramount to do well in the written section and to avoid a bare fail.

The MRCPCH Part 2 examination is divided into three parts: case histories or 'grey cases', data interpretation and visual material.

Particular care should be paid to the phrasing of answers.
Abbreviations should be avoided.

- Where a choice is allowed the most relevant investigation should be listed first.
- Poor wording may lose vital marks in this close-marked exam.

Case Histories

- There are five of these with unequal weighting.
- The first question is common to the adult MRCP paper and thus usually involves a problem of adolescence such as diabetes, Guillain-Barré etc.
- Neonatology questions are now always represented and require some practical experience of neonatal intensive care.

Data Interpretation

- Ten questions are presented.
- ECGs, EEGs, family trees and audiograms are included.

Visual material

These are mostly clinical photographs, although less than half may consist of radiological imaging, blood films etc.

The Future

Since the first edition of this book the Royal College of Paediatrics and Child Health has been established. The MRCPCH Part 1 examination will be run independently by this new college from May 1999. The requirement for candidates to pass Part 2 within seven years of success at Part 1 remains. The restriction of six attempts at Part 2 will be lifted. The first joint Part 2 examination will be available in January 1999. Candidates taking Part 2 between this date and the last sitting of 2003 will have the option of applying for the award of MRCP (UK) Diploma or the MRPCH Diploma. There is talk of different marking schemes and a move away from the competitive pass rates in the Part 2 written paper, to more criterion referenced tests. The authors believe that although the exam is unlikely to become easier, it will become fairer and more relevant to paediatricians. This is a good thing and long overdue.

About this book

Questions have been set out in the form of seven individual papers with accompanying rubric. Visual material has again been omitted, as there are a growing number of excellent atlases. All manner of imaging studies now accompany our everyday clinical work and could be an item on the paper. The candidate should be familiar with X-rays, CT scans, MRI imaging and radioisotope studies. Key points in discriminating information are given and a discussion section outlines current opinion and practice. The explanations aim to provide frameworks for problem solving and pattern recognition. Most of the standard paediatric textbooks can be used to compliment the material in this book. For those candidates who want more details and have time we have included references for the 'grey' cases. These represent the most current and comprehensive review articles that summarise both the topic discussed and the available literature.

Once again we have not attempted to simulate a 'scoring system' for a number of reasons. In the exam itself the scoring system is variable and unpredictable. Some questions have only one correct answer, although others have a 'most likely diagnosis'. In the official exam rubric it states 'the correct answer will receive maximum marks; other possible diagnosis will score a lower mark'.

Where the 'best' answer is much better than others, the difference in marking between the best and other answers will be greater. There is always a 'best' answer and as this is a practice book the candidate's aim should be to achieve just that. Other relevant differential diagnoses are discussed as Key points or discussions, but perhaps unlike real life, in the exam and in this book only one answer will do.

There is a new chapter on one method of learning for the exam. We have Dr Kevin Appleton to thank for this section. None of us have any memory of ever being taught how to revise for written medical examinations. Perhaps things would have been easier if we had understood 'Mind-Mapping' then. It may not suit everyone but we recommend you give it a try.

Paul Gringras
Deb Pal
Michael Greenberg

MIND MAPS

What are mind maps and how can they help with the exam?

You will already be aware of your strengths and weaknesses when it comes to learning for exams. You will probably use techniques which you have (successfully) used over the years. Successful techniques allow you to structure, organise and integrate new information with the knowledge you already possess in order to make learning meaningful. This is important, particularly with the Part II exam, as it is a practical impossibility to read through everything again in the few days before the exam. It is important to focus on key facts, so that you may concentrate on these in order to reduce the amount of reading required when the work is revised.

Common and effective techniques to help you reduce the quantity of information you have to learn include writing short summary notes or using highlighter pens to focus on key facts. Another less common method is mind mapping. This is not an approach that everyone will find intuitively appealing, however some people find it to be a very helpful way of organising and learning information.

Mind maps are colourful, branching pictures or diagrams that can help your memory, thinking and organisation of ideas and information. They can make study more efficient by condensing facts onto a single sheet, so that very large amounts of information may be revised quickly. In Mind Map 1 (see below) the assessment and treatment of renal failure is covered, together with the ways pre-renal failure can present. To maximise the effectiveness of mind maps it is necessary to produce your own, so that each sub-heading of the mind map will trigger off associated pieces of information in your own memory. If you had Mind Map 1 in front of you during a grey case, data interpretation or clinical viva, you would be able to answer most questions on this topic.

Mind maps work by increasing the cross connections and associations of stored material in your memory. They use images or key words to anchor information and to trigger associations. It is possible to hold entire mind maps in visual memory using this method and they make learning more enjoyable and revision less tedious. By using different modes of memory storage (e.g. factual, visual and colour), they increase the modalities and ways in which information can be stored; linear text uses only one such modality.

How to create your own mind maps

It is better to draw mind maps across the horizontal axis of the page as the structure spreads out better this way. Start with a central image or icon. Recalling this from visual memory will trigger your recall of the whole map. Next, arrange main headings or key words around this from the centre of the page. Subheadings, lists and further details can then be added to each branch.

One heading or icon in your mind will come to represent many other responses. These act as anchors for surrounding text and help you to recall this additional information efficiently. Well organised information should result in an aesthetically pleasing map; poorly organised information will look a mess and will not be recalled as well. To structure the content clearly on paper means that it must also be structured clearly in your mind so that drawing out the diagram is itself an effective means of revision. Although computer programs are now available to standardise the method, it is perhaps the actual practice of putting different coloured pens on paper, combined with your own 'aide memoires' which contribute to the whole learning process.

Because mind maps can summarise large amounts of data into a manageable form, this information can be reviewed very quickly just before the exam, maximising the 'recency' effect. Colleagues have found that in the 48 hours before the written paper they were able to review the entire syllabus which had been summarised into mind maps.

A full account of the use of mind maps can be found in 'The Mind Map Book' by Tony Busan.

Dr Kevin Appleton

Reference

The Mind Map Book, Busan T, Busan B, BBC Books, London, (1993).

We acknowledge WB Saunders Company Ltd for the use of this chapter.

Mind Map: Acute Renal Failure

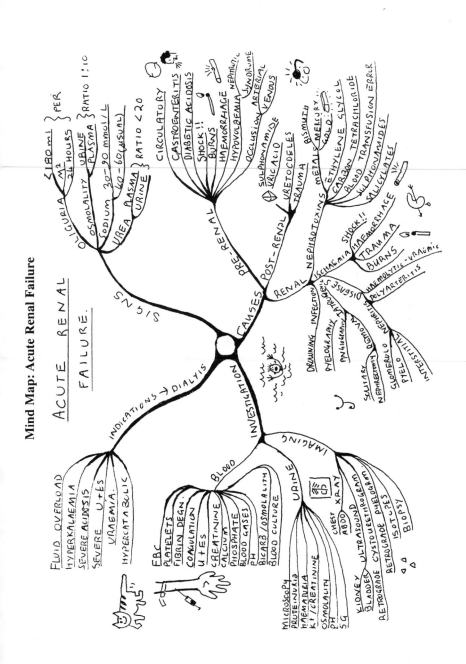

NORMAL RANGES AND ROUTINE VALUES

This list is by no means intended to replace any of the available lists of normal values and is not comprehensive.

There are, however, various values that the candidate will be expected to know since normal ranges are not provided.

Past questions, for example, have expected the candidate's knowledge of the physiological fall in haemoglobin towards the second week. Other questions have depended on knowledge of normal cerebrospinal fluid indices in the neonate.

HAEMATOLOGICAL VALUES:

AGE	Hb(g/dl)	PCV	MCV(fl)	MCHC(g/dl)	WCC(10^9/l)
Cord blood	13.5–20.0	0.50–0.56	110–128	29.5–33.5	9–30
14 days	14.5–18.0	0.50–0.58	107–121	31–34	6–15
One year	10.5–13.0	0.36–0.40	80–96	32–36	6–15

Serum Iron: 5–25 micromoles/l infants
                10–30 micromoles/l children
Ferritin: up to 150 micrograms/l in children
B_{12}:   150–1000 nanograms/l
Folate: 3.0-20 nanograms/l

Haemostatic Values:
Platelet count: 150–400 10^9/l
Bleeding time: up to 6 mins
Prothrombin time: within 2–3 seconds of control (INR ~ 1)
Partial thromboplastin time: within 6–7 seconds of control

BIOCHEMICAL RANGES

Sodium: 132–145 mmol/l
Potassium: neonate 4.0–7.0
             child 3.5–5.5 mmol/l
Urea: 2.5–8.0 mmol/l
Calcium: neonate 1.8–2.8 mmol/l
             child 2.15–2.70 mmol/l

Phosphate: neonate 1.3–3.0 mmol/l
               child 1.0–1.8 mmol/l
Osmolality: 275–295 mOsmol/kg
Thyroxine: infant 90–200 mmol/l
               child 65–180 mmol/l
Thyroid stimulating hormone: child up to 5mU/l

URINE
Osmolality greater than 870 mOsm/kg after overnight fluid deprivation

CSF

Glucose: 2.5–4.5 mmol/l (Need blood glucose to interpret, should be
              around 75% of blood glucose)
Protein: newborn 0.4–1.2 (g/l)
              neonate 0.2–0.8
              child 0.15–0.45

Mean values of non-infected CSF in young infants*		
CSF fluid parameter	0–4 weeks	4–8 weeks
Leucocyte count (/mm^3)	11.0	7.1
Polymorphs (/mm^3)	2	3
Absolute neutrophil count (/mm^3)	0.4	0.2

*ref: Bonadio WA, Bruce R, Barry D, Smith D
       Paediatric Infectious Disease Journal 1992, 11:589–591

CASE HISTORY PAPER

(Time available: 55 minutes)

1. Answer **all the questions** based upon the following 5 case histories in the spaces provided.

2. When asked (for example) to list 3 diagnoses or investigations, one line will be provided for each answer. If more than the required number of answers are given, the additional answers will not be scored.

Case History 1

A 14 year old girl is investigated for short stature. She was diagnosed as having anorexia nervosa two years ago, soon after her menarche. Since then, despite behavioural and family therapy she has remained anorexic and has been amenorrhoeic for the last year.

On examination she is very thin with dry lips and angular cheilitis. Examination of other systems normal. Blood pressure normal. Urinalysis normal.

Hb 9.9 g/dl
WBC 12.1 x 10^9/l
Platelets 320 x 10^9/l
ESR 40 mm/hr
Na 136 mmol/l
K 3.6 mmol/l
Urea 3.1 mmol/l

Question 1

a) What further investigation would be useful in making a diagnosis?

....

b) What is the most likely diagnosis?

....

Case History 2

A baby is born prematurely at 34 weeks' gestation. He is normal at birth then vomits and at 12 hours is tachypnoeic. Feeds are stopped and he settles with nasogastric feeding. At 3 days of age he becomes apnoeic, is intubated and ventilated. Jerking movements are noted whilst on the ventilator.

Investigations:
  Urea and electrolytes normal
  Blood glucose 2.4 mmol/l
  HCO_3 10 mmol/l
  pH 7.1
  FiO_2 0.28
  PaO_2 10 kPa (arterial)
  $PaCO_2$ 5.1 kPa (arterial
  Base excess = -17 mmol/l
  Chest X-ray normal
  CSF protein 1.4 g/l, glucose 1.9 mmol/l
  CSF WBC 28/mm^3, polymorphs, RBC 44/mm^3
  CSF Gram stain no organisms seen

Cerebral ultrasound shows diffusely increased echogenicity, the ventricles are not clearly seen.

Question 2

a) What is the most useful investigation?

  ....

b) What is the most likely diagnosis?

  ....

Case History 3

A nine year old boy presents with a two week history of an unproductive cough and pain over the right chest wall. He has been treated for right lower lobe pneumonia with ampicillin for one week and co-trimoxazole for four days. The child is getting worse with a poor appetite and weight loss, headache and dizziness.

Father is a postman. His mother had pneumonia responding to antibiotics two weeks ago. His seven year old brother is well and the family lives in a two room council flat with a cat and a budgie.

On examination he is pyrexial 40°C and looks ill. Pulse rate 170. He appears mildly dehydrated with signs of recent weight loss. There is reduced movement of the right side of the chest, dull percussion note and reduced breath sounds in the right lower zone accompanied by crepitations. The rest of the examination is normal. Urinalysis is negative.

Investigations:
Hb 10.9 g/dl   WBC 6.2 x 10^9/l diff. normal ESR 65 mm/hr
Reticulocytes 3.5% MCHC 33 g/dl
Sputum culture   mixed growth
Mantoux test   negative
Chest X-ray   Right lower lobe consolidation
                 Right costophrenic effusion
Pleural tap   1 ml clear serous fluid, 2 WBC: culture negative

Question 3

a) What investigations are of most value in diagnosis?

....

....

....

b) What is the drug of choice?

....

Case History 4

A 13 year old boy presents with a 3 day history of productive cough with purulent sputum. On several occasions, the cough produced a cupful of bright red blood.

He was well until 2 months previously when he was struck in the chest whilst playing football. He remained breathless for a few hours before recovering.

Two days later whilst sitting at his school desk he had a sudden paroxysm of severe coughing which eventually settled, so he was well on returning home.

One week later he described symptoms of right sided pleuritic chest pain and a cough productive of small amounts of mucoid sputum, stained with flecks of blood.

He was seen in hospital, at that stage apyrexial with a normal white blood count and negative blood cultures. Chest X-ray showed patchy infiltration of the right lower lobe. He was treated with oral erythromycin and responded well clinically and radiologically.

Two weeks later he was admitted again. This time his temperature was 38.5°C, he had bronchial breathing and crackles at the right lung base. The chest X-ray demonstrated consolidation with a possible fluid level in the posterior segment of the right lower lobe.

Question 4

a) What is the most likely diagnosis?

....

b) What is the most important investigation?

....

Case History 5

A two and a half year old caucasian boy was admitted with a history of diarrhoea and abdominal pain.

Over the last three weeks he had been mildly unwell with a cough and cold which had improved over the previous week. Two days prior to admission he had watery green diarrhoea, the last three stools being flecked with fresh blood. The abdominal pain was constant but worse on opening his bowels causing him to cry and draw his knees up.

In the past he had had a tonsillectomy and required tympanostomy for chronic serous otitis media five months previously. His only medication was cough linctus.

On examination he was apyrexial, tired and miserable. He was not clinically dehydrated. Abdomen was generally tender but soft with no palpable masses. The rest of the examination was normal.

Investigations:
Hb 12.3 g/dl
WBC 21.9 x 10^9/l
Platelets 737 x 10^9/l
Na 135 mmol/l
K 4.1 mmol/l
HCO_3 18 mmol/l
Urea 6.9 mmol/l
Creatinine 73 mmol/l
Glucose 4.5 mmol/l

Blood cultures and stool specimens were sent for culture and he was commenced on maintenance intravenous fluids. The next day he continued to have abdominal pain and pass bloody mucous stools. A plain abdominal X-ray with the appearance of fluid levels was followed by a normal barium enema examination.

On the fourth day of admission with no improvement he was noted not to have passed urine for twelve hours. He looked pale and unwell, with slight puffiness of the eyelids and mildly jaundiced sclerae. A fluid challenge was unsuccessful.

Investigations:
Na 124 mmol/l
K 5.5 mmol/l
HCO3 19 mmol/l
Urea 12.6 mmol/l
Creatinine 163 mmol/l

Question 5

a) What immediate investigation would you perform?

....

b) What additional clinical information is required?

....

c) What is the most likely explanation for the deterioration?

....

EXAM 1

DATA INTERPRETATION PAPER

(Time available: 45 minutes)

1. Answer **all 10 of the following questions** in the spaces provided.

2. When asked (for example) to list 3 diagnoses or investigations, one line will be provided for each answer. If more than the required number of answers are given, the additional answers will not be scored.

Question 1

A 12 year old African boy is tested for sickle cell disease pre-operatively. His father is known to have sickle cell trait.

Results   Hb 10.1 g/dl
RBC 6.1 x 10^{12}/l
MCV 65 fl
MCH 21.1 pg
MCHC 30 g/dl
Sickle test positive
HbS 71%
HbA 21.5%
HbA2 4.5%
HbF 3%
Serum ferritin 159 mcg/l

a) What haemoglobinopathy does the boy have?

....

b) What haemoglobinopathy would you expect on testing the mother?

....

Question 2

A boy has the following blood results:

Ca 2.4 mmol/l   PO4 0.7 mmol/l   Alkaline Phosphatase 510 u/l
Parathyroid hormone normal   25(OH)D3 normal   Creatinine normal
Urine pH normal, no glycosuria, no aminociduria

a) What is the diagnosis?

....

Question 3

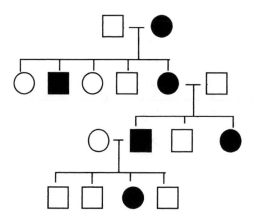

a) What is the mode of inheritance shown?

....

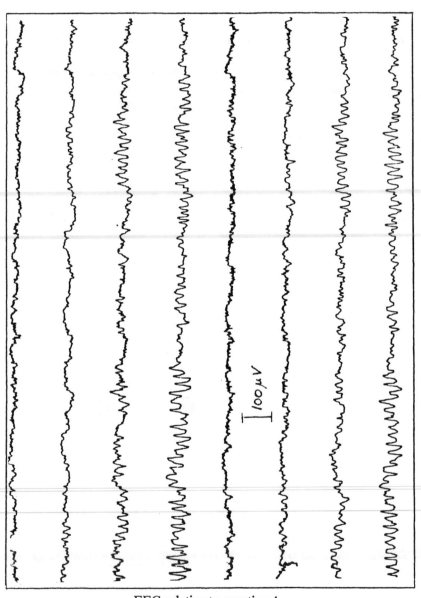

EEG relating to question 4

Question 4

This 12 year old schoolboy is under investigation for frequent 'faints', often occurring early in the morning, and episodes of poor concentration at school. He is right handed and the EEG shown opposite was performed while he was awake.

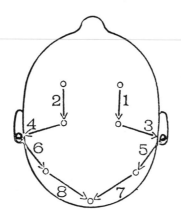

Montage Used

a) What does this EEG show?

    ....

Question 5

A 9 month old boy is admitted for investigation of failure to thrive and persistent chest infections.

Investigations:
   Hb 9.1 g/dl
   WBC 12.4 x 10^9/l
   Platelets 260 x 10^9/l
   Na 126 mmol/l
   K 2.0 mmol/l
   Cl 82 mmol/l
   Urea 4.0 mmol/l
   HCO_3 40 mmol/l

Sweat test
   Weight of sweat collected 200 mg
   Na 75 mmol/l
   Cl 82 mmol/l
   K 40 mmol/l

a) What is the diagnosis?

   ....

b) Describe the electrolyte abnormalities.

   ....

c) What is the cause of these abnormalities?

   ....

Question 6

An 11 year old boy performed standard spirometry and produced the following results:

	Actual value	Predicted value
FVC (l)	1.13	2.07
FEV_1(l)	1.08	1.87
FEV_1/FVC (%)	95	97
FEF 25-75% (l/sec)	1.89	2.26

a) What type of respiratory impairment is present?

....

b) Give three possible causes for these results.

....

....

....

Question 7

A boy can do the following:

- hold a cup with both hands
- speak in two to three word sentences
- walk up stairs with one hand held
- after several attempts, build a three block tower

a) What is his developmental age?

....

Question 8

A 4 year old girl has a cardiac catheter investigation:

Site	O_2 Saturation(%)	Pressure (mmHg)
SVC	75	4
IVC	74	
RA	75	
RV	90	90/8
PA	90	20/4
LA	90	6
LV	89	92/10
Aorta	80	90/50

a) What two abnormalities are present?

    ....

    ....

b) What is the most likely diagnosis?

    ....

Question 9

Examine the audiogram below.

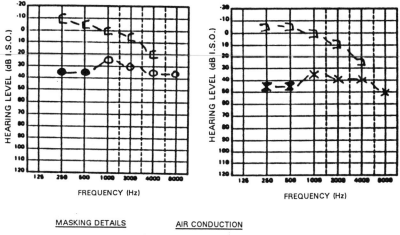

MASKING DETAILS — AIR CONDUCTION

RIGHT	O	LEFT	X
MASKED	●	MASKED	✕

BONE CONDUCTION

UNMASKED (RIGHT OR LEFT) ▲

MASKED RIGHT [LEFT]

a) What does it show?

....

b) Give a possible cause for this.

....

Question 10

A 6 day old baby boy was born weighing 3.95 kg. After some mild temperature fluctuation on the first day he is discharged home the following day. On the third day he is readmitted looking very ill and lethargic. He is resuscitated with plasma. Serum electrolytes on admission were as follows:

Na 132 mmol/l
K 4.7 mmol/l
Bilirubin 320 μmol/l
Weight 3.4 kg
Urine osmolality 88 mOsm/kg

a) What further investigation needs to be performed?

....

More detailed studies are carried out:

Serum 17 hydroxy progesterone 2.6 nmol/l (normal < 20 nmol/l)
Plasma renin   high
Plasma aldosterone   low
Plasma ACTH   very high
Plasma cortisol   96 nmol/l

Urine Na   90 mmol/l
24 hour urine steroid profile
    androgens   very low
    cortisol metabolites   very low

b) What is the diagnosis?

....

c) How would you treat the child after initial resuscitation?

....

CASE HISTORY PAPER

(Time available: 55 minutes)

1. Answer **all the questions** based upon the following 5 case histories in the spaces provided.

2. When asked (for example) to list 3 diagnoses or investigations, one line will be provided for each answer. If more than the required number of answers are given, the additional answers will not be scored.

Case History 1

A 2 year old girl is brought into casualty having become unsteady an hour before, then very agitated and arching her back.

Her birth history and past medical history are normal. Her parents were away for the weekend and she was staying with her grandmother, who enjoyed looking after her since the recent death of her husband.

On initial examination there were no focal neurological signs, her temperature was 35.5°C and other systems were normal. Subsequently, whilst still in the casualty department, she had three convulsions, affecting the arms and legs symmetrically, each lasting about three minutes.

Investigations:
    Na 135 mmol/l
    K 3.8 mmol/l
    Urea 2.6 mmol/l
    Glucose 5.1 mmol/l
    Ca 2.3 mmol/l
    Albumin 38 mmol/l

    CSF   RBC $1 \times 10^6/l$
             WBC $4 \times 10^6/l$
             glucose 4.0 mmol/l
             protein 390 mg/l

Question 1

a) What is the diagnosis?

....

b) What is the prognosis?

....

Case History 2

A 12 year old boy presented with a 2 month history of malaise and weight loss. He had previously been well with no significant past medical history.

He and his family were from Pakistan and the patient had last visited there when he was 10 years old.

His father had a history of asthma and renal stones but otherwise there was no significant family history.

On examination he was thin and febrile 38.5°C. There was no cyanosis or clubbing and his JVP was seen at the level of his jaw. His respiratory rate was 28 per minute and on auscultation, his breath sounds were vesicular. Pulse 85, apex beat not palpable, heart sounds normal. Abdominal examination revealed a 3 cm enlarged, smooth and non-tender liver. Ascites was present, no other masses palpable.

Investigations:
Hb 12.1
WBC 6.4 x 10^9/l polymorphs 60%
lymphocytes 25%
eosinophils 6%
basophils 6%

ALT 15   Albumin 34   Bilirubin 24
Prothrombin time 15/12

Mantoux negative at 1 in 10,000

Peritoneal aspirate:
Protein   28 g/l
Glucose   5.4 mmol/l
no cells

CXR: heart size normal, no abnormalities seen

Question 2

a) What two investigations would you do next?

....

....

b) What is the most likely diagnosis?

....

Case History 3

A 9 day old baby boy is admitted with a two day history of diarrhoea and vomiting.

His birth had been normal, birth weight 3.7 kg at term, and initially had bottle fed well. Both parents had recently had viral gastroenteritis.

Whilst in hospital, intravenous fluids were commenced since he continued to vomit. Initial urine microscopy showed haematuria and he became oliguric during the course of the day. Ten hours after admission he had two short generalised convulsions.

On examination he looked pale and clinically dehydrated. He disliked abdominal examination, screaming and drawing his legs up to his chest. A mass was palpable in the right hypochondrium. The rest of the examination was normal.

Investigations:
Hb 16 g/dl
WBC 22 x 10^9/l (70% neutrophils)
Platelets 35 x 10^9/l

Blood urea 28 mmol/l

Question 3

a) What is the most likely diagnosis?

....

b) Name three useful confirmatory investigations.

....

....

....

c) Give three possible causes for the convulsions.

....

....

....

Case History 4

A 4 month old boy presents with diarrhoea since birth, tachypnoea and a seborrhoeic skin rash. There is no palpable lymphadenopathy. Two siblings died at age one week and four weeks with diarrhoea.

Investigation:
Chest X-ray interstitial shadowing
Hb 11.0 g/dl
WBC 5.1 x 10^9/l
Eosinophils 35%
Platelets 255 x 10^9/l
IgA absent
IgG low
IgM low

Question 4

a) What is the underlying disease?

....

b) What organism is the likely cause of the pneumonia?

....

c) What is the best treatment for the pneumonia?

....

Case History 5

A two year old boy presents with recurrent convulsions. He was born by forceps delivery at 2.4 kg. His development has been normal and his immunisations up to date. His parents are both 25 years old and well although father suffered fits until the age of three. The four year old sister is well.

His first attack occurred six months ago following an upper respiratory tract infection associated with fever. Four more attacks have occurred, all in the early morning. The child is said to be irritable before breakfast and possibly a little unsteady on his feet. He is well in between attacks and takes phenobarbitone 30 mg bd.

On examination he is alert and looks healthy. His height and weight are both below the 3rd centile. There is a 3 cm smooth non-tender hepatomegaly but otherwise examination is normal.

Urinalysis is normal.

Investigations:
Na 138 mmol/l
K 4.5 mmol/l
Urea 4.0 mmol/l
Ca 2.25 mmol/l
PO_4 1.2 mmol/l
Alkaline Phosphatase 800 IU
Fasting glucose 1.6 mmol/l
Hb 11.9 g/dl
WBC 6.4 x 10^9/l
Bone age 18 months

Question 5

a) What is the most likely diagnosis?

....

b) What investigation would you do to confirm the diagnosis?

....

EXAM 2

DATA INTERPRETATION PAPER

(Time available: 45 minutes)

1. Answer **all 10 of the following questions** in the spaces provided.

2. When asked (for example) to list 3 diagnoses or investigations, one line will be provided for each answer. If more than the required number of answers are given, the additional answers will not be scored.

Question 1

A 4 year old Indian girl presents with a 4 day history of increasing puffiness around the eyes. Investigations are as follows:

Na 136 mmol/l
K 5.2 mmol/l
Urea 8.1 mmol/l
Protein 42 g/dl
Albumin 26 g/dl
Hb 12.6 g/dl
WBC 10.2 x 10^9/l
Platelets 170 x 10^9/l
Urinalysis pH 6.5
protein + + +
trace blood

a) What is the most likely diagnosis?

....

b) Give four further investigations.

....

....

....

....

c) Outline management in two sentences.

....

....

....

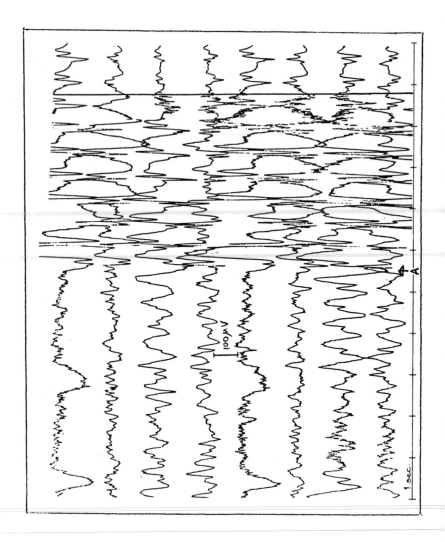

EEG relating to question 2

Question 2

A 6 year old girl is reported by her teacher to have episodic staring spells. During these her facial expression is statue-like and she blinks her eyes. Her physical examination is normal and her EEG is shown opposite.

a) What is the diagnosis?

....

b) What manoeuvre may have been performed at point A?

....

c) Would you perform any further neurological investigations before commencing treatment?

....

Question 3

A baby girl is investigated for prolonged neonatal jaundice. The glucose 6 phosphate dehydrogenase level is found to be subnormal. In addition the mother's G6PD is marginally low whilst father's is normal.

What is the chance of finding a normal G6PD in

a) a male sibling?

....

b) a female sibling?

....

Question 4

A 6 year old boy is investigated for growth failure. Two years previously he had a course of radiotherapy for a medulloblastoma.

Insulin tolerance test

Time (mins)	0	20	30	60	90	120
Glucose (mmol/l)	4.5	1.8	1.6	6.3	7.5	8.1
Cortisol (nmol/l)	508		581	992	741	582
GH (mU/l)	0.9		0.7	1.7	4.2	4.6
TSH (mU/l)	41	>60		>60		
FSH U/l	1.6	>30		>30		
LH U/l	1.2	2.8		3.2		

a) What are the causes of his growth failure?

....

....

....

Question 5

A 10 month old boy from Kenya is referred with failure to thrive. He weighs 4.1 kg and was apparently a normal baby. He is able to sit up if gently supported. He cannot yet crawl or pull himself to standing. He has suffered recurrent otitis media in the last two months despite antibiotic treatment.

Investigations:
Hb 8.9 g/dl
WBC 16 x 10^9/l   PMN 50%
lymphocytes 40%
monocytes 6%
eosinophils 1%

ESR 15 mm/h

Sickle test negative
Albumin 23 g/l

Immunoglobulins   IgG 410 iu/ml (35-115)
IgM 236 iu/ml (35-185)
IgA 96 iu/ml (10-65)

a) What is the probable diagnosis?

....

b) What two tests may help to confirm this diagnosis?

....

....

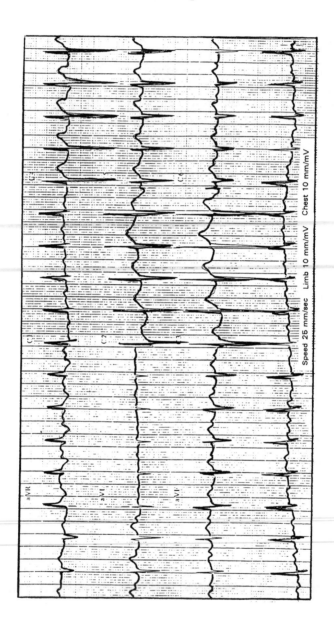

<u>ECG relating to question 6</u>

Question 6

a) Describe three features in the ECG.

....

....

....

b) What is the diagnosis?

....

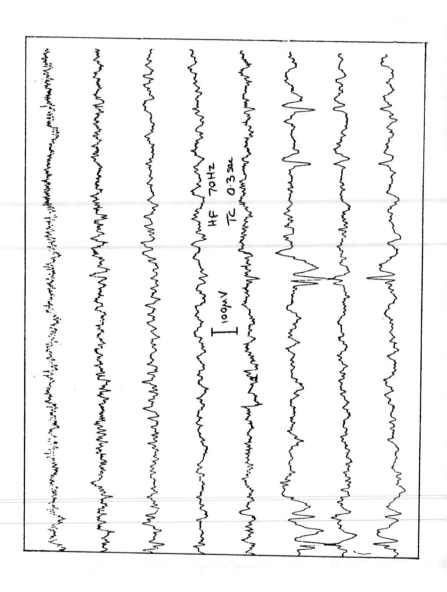

EEG relating to question 7

Question 7

A 9 year old boy is thought to be having night terrors. He has been waking up two hours after falling asleep, making guttural sounds, and one side of his face twitches for about a minute. During this time he understands what is said to him but cannot speak intelligibly. His EEG is shown opposite.

a) Describe any EEG abnormality.

....

b) What is the diagnosis?

....

Question 8

A child with a one-week history of febrile illness treated with ampicillin presents with mild neck stiffness and hemiplegia. CSF results are given:

CSF protein 0.8 g/l
CSF glucose 0.7 mmol/l
CSF WBC 300/mm^3, 68% lymphocytes

Peripheral blood WBC 15 x 10^9/l, 58% lymphocytes

a) What is the diagnosis?

....

Question 9

A 28 week preterm baby is being ventilated for respiratory distress syndrome. The baby is sedated and the ventilator is set at:

Rate   50/min
Pressure   20/3
I:E ratio   1:1
FiO_2 0.8

Arterial blood gases are:

pH   7.15
PaO_2 6.4 kPa
$PaCO_2$ 7.5 kPa
Base excess   -7.1 mmol/l

a) List two ways to improve the ventilation.

....

....

Question 10

A girl with a history of recurrent urinary tract infections presents with renal colic. The plain abdominal X-ray shows calculi in the renal tract.

Na 132 mmol/l
K 3.1 mmol/l
Cl 114 mmol/l
Urea 12 mmol/l

arterial pH 7.23
urine pH 6.6

a) What is the likely diagnosis?

....

b) Give three possible causes.

....

....

....

c) Give two treatment measures.

....

....

EXAM 3

CASE HISTORY PAPER

(Time available: 55 minutes)

1. Answer **all the questions** based upon the following 5 case histories in the spaces provided.

2. When asked (for example) to list 3 diagnoses or investigations, one line will be provided for each answer. If more than the required number of answers are given, the additional answers will not be scored.

Case History 1

A 12 year old schoolboy was seen with lower back pain. It began 3 weeks ago during a school P. E. lesson. He initially stayed in bed but despite rest still complained of continual pain. He found walking painful and seemed unsteady on his feet.

His throat had been sore for the past week and his appetite poor. Although he had no dysuria, he complained of frequency and occasional incontinence of urine.

He has been previously well apart from a prolonged chest infection when 10 years old.

On examination he looks unwell, pyrexial 38.0°C. Pale conjunctivae. There is a large unexplained bruise on the right thigh. His throat is red and there are several cervical glands palpable. An enlarged non-tender node is palpable in the left axilla. His back and neck are very stiff, all movements are limited. There is increased tone in both legs. The right ankle jerk is absent but the other tendon reflexes are normal. There is decreased sensation over the dorsum of the right foot.

Question 1

a) What is the most likely diagnosis?

....

b) What two investigations would help confirm the diagnosis?

....

....

Case History 2

A baby is born at 30 weeks gestation and develops respiratory distress syndrome. On day 2 he requires pressures of 24/4, I:E ratio 1:1 and rate of 30 per minute. Blood gas results are satisfactory. Four hours later his clinical condition deteriorates, despite having looking well a few minutes earlier.

Appropriate action is taken and five minutes later the baby is looking well again.

Question 2

a) Give four possible complications of management which may account for the rapid deterioration and recovery.

....

....

....

....

Case History 3

A 6 year old boy is seen by his school doctor. For the last two months he has been off games because of pain in his knees. He has been well before this apart from a fever and headaches two or three months ago. He is fully immunised and has two sisters who are well. His parents are divorced and his mother, whom he lives with, is a fashion designer. She has a history of alcoholism but claims to have been abstinent for three years. The boy is taking 0.5% hydrocortisone cream for a spreading patch of eczema on his trunk and paracetamol for occasional headaches. On questioning, he admits to no particular difficulties at school. His hobbies include constructing aircraft models.

On examination he is shy and pale. Pulse 88, chest and heart normal. Abdomen is soft with 2 cm liver edge palpable on deep inspiration. Both knees appear normal on inspection but slightly painful at the limits of movement. His gait is normal but he finds it difficult to run. The other joints are normal. There is a sacral dimple and, at the waist, an 8 cm erythematous ring with a faded patch in the centre. There is no bruising evident.

Question 3

a) What additional element of the history would you like to elicit?

....

b) How would you make the diagnosis?

....

c) What is your management?

....

....

Case History 4

An 8 year old child with cystic fibrosis presents with gradual onset of generalised abdominal pain and bile stained vomiting over the last two days.

On examination 5% dehydrated, apyrexial. Abdomen moderately distended with generalised tenderness but no guarding. There is a firm mass in the right iliac fossa. The rectum is empty on examination but a mass is palpable in the right iliac fossa.

Question 4

a) Give three differential diagnoses.

....

....

....

b) What investigation would be most helpful?

....

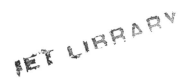

Case History 5

A 14 year old girl presents with pain in the lower back and difficulty bending down for the last three days. She thinks her face is swollen and feels weak in her arms and legs. Earlier in the day she had an episode of double vision lasting half an hour. At the age of six she suffered meningitis but made a complete recovery.

On examination she is not breathless or cyanosed. She has no neck stiffness and has an expressionless face. She is unable to close her eyes when asked. Neither can she lift her limbs off the couch. All limb reflexes are absent, the abdominal reflex is present and sensation to light touch is intact.

Investigations:
 Hb 12.6 g/dl
 WBC 5.8 x 10^9/l
 ESR 7 mm/h
 Na 134 mmol/l
 K 5.2 mmol/l
 Urea 5.5 mmol/l
 Creatinine 62 mmol/l

Question 5

a) What is the most likely diagnosis?

 ....

b) What investigation would you do next?

 ....

c) How would you monitor her progress?

 ....

EXAM 3

DATA INTERPRETATION PAPER

(Time available: 45 minutes)

1. Answer **all 10 of the following questions** in the spaces provided.

2. When asked (for example) to list 3 diagnoses or investigations, one line will be provided for each answer. If more than the required number of answers are given, the additional answers will not be scored.

Question 1

A 10 week old baby presents with a two week history of vomiting.

Na 126 mmol/l
K 3.1 mmol/l
Cl 72 mmol/l
Urea 8.4 mmol/l
pH 7.53
HCO_3 45 mmol/l
Glucose 3.6 mmol/l

a) What is the diagnosis?

....

Question 2

Family tree showing affected boy with achondroplasia, normal sister and normal parents.

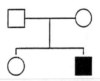

a) What is the risk of a further child being affected?

....

b) What is the risk of the sibling having an affected child?

....

Question 3

A 10 month old obese child presents with hypoglycaemia. There is no ketonuria.

Investigations:
    Serum triglycerides raised
    Serum cholesterol raised
    Plasma glucose (random)   3.0 mmol/l   insulin 25 IU
    Plasma glucose (fasting)   1.8 mmol/l   insulin 4.0 IU

a) What is the diagnosis?

    ....

Question 4

An 11 year old boy with cystic fibrosis complained of a wheeze on exertion. Lung function tests were performed before and 20 minutes after nebulised salbutamol 5 mg:

	Pre	*Post*	*Expected*
Forced vital capacity (l)	1.7	1.8	2.1
FEV_1 (l)	1.0	1.5	1.81
Residual volume (l)	1.1	0.9	0.75
Total lung capacity (l)	3.3	3.1	3.0

a) List the three physiological abnormalities these results demonstrate.

....

....

....

b) Name two laboratory techniques that can be employed to measure these lung volumes.

....

....

Question 5

A 13 year old girl is brought for consultation by her mother who believes the girl is not growing. Assessment shows her weight to be increasing satisfactorily and her height to be below the third centile. Her height velocity is falling and she has not entered puberty. Her bone age is 8.28 years.

a) What two investigations would you consider next?

....

....

Combined pituitary function tests are shown below.

Time (mins)	0	20	30	60	90	120
Glucose mmol/l	4.1	0.9	2.1	6.5	8.1	8.7
Cortisol nmol/l	337		797	868	710	640
GH mU/l	0.9		1.4	11.6	4.5	1.0
TSH mU/l	>60	59		>60		
FSH U/l	2.3	6.1		15		
LH U/l	2.0	3.9		45		
PrL mU/l	580	3000		1980		

b) What is the diagnosis?

....

c) How would you treat her and what would you advise the parents?

....

....

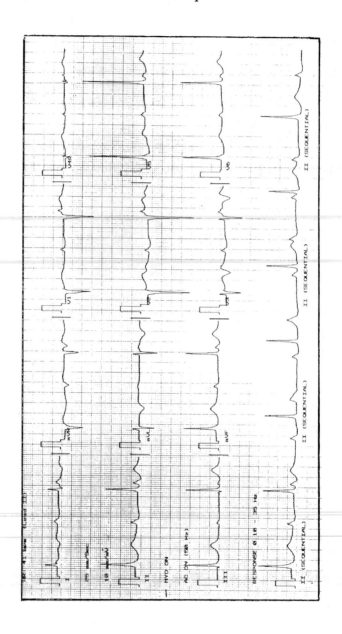

ECG relating to question 6

Question 6

a) What diagnosis can be made from the ECG shown opposite?

....

Question 7

A 7 year old girl with haematuria and purpura has the following blood results:

Hb 6.8 g/dl
WBC 5.0 x 10^9/l
Platelets 15 x 10^9/l

a) Give two possible diagnoses.

....

....

Question 8

A 5 month old infant presents with a vague history of malaise, lethargy and fever for two weeks. On examination he has a macular rash over the body, his hands are slightly oedematous and peeling. His tonsils are enlarged and he has some large lymph nodes in the neck.

Hb 11.1 g/dl
WBC 24.0 x 10^9/l
Platelets 980 x 10^9/l
Na 133 mmol/l
K 4.5 mmol/l
HCO_3 18 mmol/l
Urea 3.5 mmol/l
Throat swab no growth
ASOT normal

a) What is the most important differential diagnosis?

....

b) What investigations need to be performed?

....

c) What, if any, treatment should be commenced?

....

Question 9

A boy is asked to copy shapes. He is able to copy a circle and a cross but not a square. When asked to count as far as he can he reaches three. He knows his first name but not his surname.

a) How old is he?

    ....

b) What would you do next?

    ....

Question 10

A well 8 week old baby is referred because of pallor noticed in a routine 6 week development clinic. This is the mother's second child and the neonatal period was uneventful.

Investigations:
   Mother's blood group A NEG

   Cord blood
       Hb 16.2 g/dl
       WBC $10.1 \times 10^9/l$
       Platelets $261 \times 10^9/l$
       group O pos
       DAT NEG

   at 8 weeks
   Hb 5.1 g/dl
   WBC $12.4 \times 10^9/l$
   Platelets $321 \times 10^9/l$

a) Name the three most useful investigations.

   ....

   ....

   ....

b) What is the most likely diagnosis?

   ....

CASE HISTORY PAPER

(Time available 55 minutes)

1. Answer **all the questions** based upon the following 5 case histories in the spaces provided.

2. When asked (for example) to list 3 diagnoses or investigations, one line will be provided for each answer. If more than the required number of answers are given, the additional answers will not be scored.

Case History 1

A 15 year old girl with known complex congenital heart disease is referred to the paediatrician by her general practitioner. Two weeks previously she had complained of increasing shortness of breath and was noted to have an irregular pulse. She is now experiencing chest pain and has coughed up blood stained sputum. She had a repair of her heart defect at the age of eighteen months and has had regular follow up since.

On examination she is cyanosed, has a loud second heart sound and both systolic and diastolic murmurs. Her blood pressure and the rest of the examination are normal.

Question 1

a) What complication of the original lesion has occurred?

....

b) What has precipitated the recent deterioration?

....

c) What was the likely cause of the chest pain?

....

Case History 2

The paediatrician is called to the postnatal ward to examine a six day old baby girl who is jittery and has had a low grade pyrexia over the last 24 hours.

The baby was born, weighing 3.4 kg, by forceps delivery to a 22 year old primigravida. The mother was unbooked and little antenatal history known. At present she is staying with friends in a rented flat. By her estimated dates the baby is 38 weeks gestation.

There was delay in the second stage of labour and a brief type II deceleration on the cardiotocograph trace thirty minutes prior to delivery. Apgar scores of 9 at 1 minute and 10 at 5 minutes were recorded. Since birth she has bottle fed avidly and the midwife observes that she always seems hungry and is difficult to settle to sleep.

On examination her temperature is 37.8°C, weight 3.35 kg and she sucks well. Pulse 180, no murmurs, respiratory rate 40, breath sounds normal. There is no skin rash but she feels sweaty. There are occasional tremulous movements of the arms and legs. Fontanelle is normal and neurological examination is also normal.

Question 2

a) What three immediate investigations would you perform?

....

....

....

b) What is the most likely diagnosis?

....

Case History 3

An 8 year old Bangladeshi boy is sent to hospital by his head teacher. He has been behaving oddly the previous day and today in class was unable to write and displayed jerky movements of his limbs and head. He was taunted in the playground by his friends who thought he was 'mad'. He had been well previously and had not been abroad recently. His birth, development and immunisations in the UK had been normal and he was said to be a difficult child at home. He did well at school and had lots of friends. He was one of nine children, his father a chef and his mother a housewife, living in an old council house. The rest of the family was well. A week ago he had been frightened by a violent neighbour in the street.

On examination he was a well nourished boy, apyrexial. He was fidgety and had continuous, rapid, irregular, jerky movements of the limbs, head and face. These movements ceased when asked to recite the five times table. He was fully orientated with normal higher functions. His speech was dysarthric and explosive. Cerebellar and peripheral nervous system examination was normal. No other abnormalities were found.

Investigations:
    Hb 11.2 g/dl
    WBC 10.8 x 10^9/l
    ESR 48 mm/h
    Na 135 mmol/l
    K 3.4 mmol/l
    Urea 4.3 mmol/l
    Creatinine 43 mmol/l
    HCO_3 22 mmol/l
    Ca 2.1 mmol/l
    PO_4 1.1 mmol/l
    Alkaline phosphatase 410
    AST 54
    Bilirubin 12 μmol/l

    Urinalysis negative

    Lead 1.4 μmol/l
    Toxin screen negative
    Throat swab no growth

Blood cultures no growth

ECG normal
EEG normal
CT brain normal

Question 3

a) What important investigation is missing?

   ....

b) What is the most likely diagnosis?

   ....

c) What treatment would you commence?

   ....

d) What is the prognosis for gait?

   ....

Case History 4

A baby girl 10 weeks old presents with failure to thrive. The birthweight was 2.3 kg at an ultrasound estimated gestation of 38 weeks. She had passed meconium normally at birth. Maternal health was normal during the pregnancy. The parents are both of short stature and low intelligence.

At 3 weeks she had abdominal distension and Hirschsprung's disease was proven by rectal biopsy. A myomectomy was performed at 5 weeks and the child discharged from hospital at 6 weeks. At 8 weeks the parents noted her to be constipated and refusing to feed. She has not vomited.

On examination she was pale but did not look ill. Her weight was 3.23 kg, temperature 36.4°C, pulse 110 and respiratory rate 32 per minute. She had periorbital oedema and noisy breathing, the nasal airways partially obstructed. She had a large tongue and an umbilical hernia. She was floppy, had no head control and did not smile. The liver was palpable 1 cm below the costal margin but no other organs were palpable in the abdomen.

Urinalysis was normal.

Investigations:
    Hb 10.2 g/dl
    WBC 8.3 x 10^9/l
    Chest X-ray normal

Question 4

a) What one investigation will confirm the diagnosis?

    ....

b) What factors mentioned will influence the mental prognosis?

    ....

    ....

Case History 5

A baby boy aged 6 months was readmitted into hospital. He had spent the first 6 weeks of his life in hospital because of ventricular septal defect and heart failure in the neonatal period. He was treated with digoxin, frusemide and spironolactone and his condition improved by discharge. At that stage his weight, length and head circumference were all between the 10th and 25th centile.

At home feeding time was always difficult but he had progressed to solids and no longer became breathless during feeds. At three months of age he began to have diarrhoea, described as loose and foul smelling, up to 5 times a day.

On admission the baby looked miserable and irritable. Weight (3.0 kg) and length are between the 3rd and 10th centile. He was on digoxin 40 μg daily and frusemide 2 mg bd, spironolactone 2.5 mg bd.

On examination his abdomen was slightly distended with the liver 1 cm below the costal margin. Examination of other systems was normal. Whilst in hospital he continued to have foul smelling, loose stools. Stool culture was negative. After two weeks in hospital he had failed to gain any weight.

Question 5

a) What is the most likely cause of his failure to thrive?

....

b) What is the best investigation to confirm the diagnosis?

....

EXAM 4

DATA INTERPRETATION

(Time available: 45 minutes)

1. Answer **all 10 of the following questions** in the spaces provided.

2. When asked (for example) to list 3 diagnoses or investigations, one line will be provided for each answer. If more than the required number of answers are given, the additional answers will not be scored.

Question 1

A 3 year old girl, previously well, presents with a history of generalised oedema for the last three months, and diarrhoea over the last two months. The diarrhoea is mild and intermittent.

Investigations:
Urine protein <30 mg/24 hours
Albumin 20 g/dl
Hb 10.2 g/dl
WBC 4.1 x 10^9/l   PMN 60%
                      lymphocytes 10%
                      monocytes   30%

a) What is the diagnosis?

....

b) Give two investigations.

....

....

Question 2

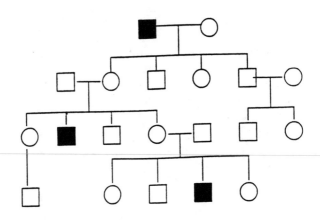

a) What is the pattern of inheritance?

....

b) What is the risk of II_3 being a carrier?

....

c) What is the risk of IV_1 being affected?

....

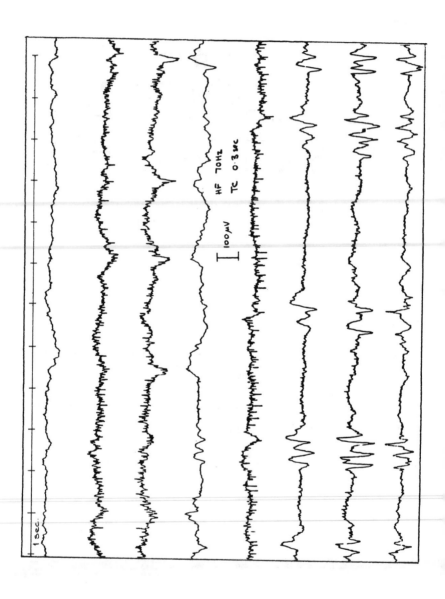

EEG relating to question 3

Question 3

a) What clinical diagnosis would be compatible with this EEG?

   ....

b) Name one cause.

   ....

Question 4

A 4 year old girl with no previous history of convulsions is admitted in status epilepticus. The following emergency investigations are performed:

Hb 7.9 g/dl
WBC 6.8 x 10^9/l
Blood glucose 4 mmol/l
Urinalysis protein + + +
Cells none seen
Casts none seen
Clinitest ¾%

a) What is the most likely diagnosis?

....

b) What three investigations would confirm this?

....

....

....

Question 5

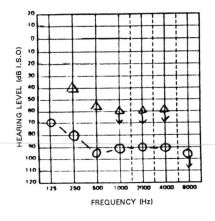 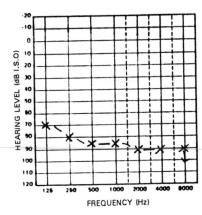

AIR CONDUCTION
RIGHT O   LEFT X

BONE CONDUCTION
UNMASKED (RIGHT OR LEFT) Δ

a) Comment on this audiogram of a 10 year old boy who had meningitis aged 3 years.

....

b) What was the most likely organism to cause this damage?

....

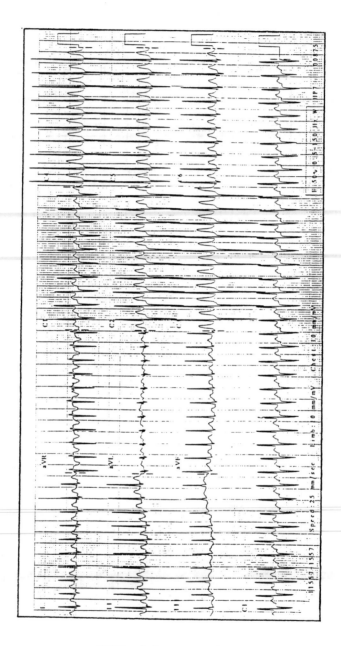

ECG relating to question 6

Question 6

a) What is the abnormality on this ECG?

....

b) How would you treat it?

....

....

Question 7

A 14 year old boy with recent onset of bilateral facial palsy following a febrile illness has this blood count:

Hb 11.2 g/dl
MCV 92 fl
MCH 32 pg
MCHC 34 g/dl
Reticulocytes 5.7%
WBC 16.2 x 10^9/l
PMN 51%
Lymphocytes 49%
Platelets 68 x 10^9/l
ESR 27 mm/h

Blood film atypical cells, spherocytes, agglutination

a) What is the underlying diagnosis?

....

b) How would you confirm this?

....

Question 8

A 6 month old girl is admitted following a febrile convulsion. On the ward she has two further generalised convulsions one hour apart, lasting 2 and 8 minutes. The second seizure is terminated by rectal diazepam.

Investigations:
Na 137 mmol/l
K 4.2 mmol/l
Urea 5.1 mmol/l
Glucose 3.6 mmol/l
Hb 12.1 g/dl
WBC 12.3 x 10^9/l
Platelets 341 x 10^9/l
CSF bloodstained
     RBC 12,000 x 10^9/l
     WBC 15 x 10^9/l
Lymphocytes 80%
Glucose 3.4 mmol/l unsuitable for protein estimation
Gram stain no organisms seen

a) What is your immediate management?

....

b) What two urgent investigations are necessary?

....

....

c) What is the likely diagnosis?

....

Question 9

A newborn baby was examined at 2 days and was found to have normal femoral pulses. On the third day he became unwell and was noted to have weak femoral pulses. The following cardiac catheterisation data were obtained:

Site	O_2 Saturation (%)	Pressure (mmHg)
SVC	55	8
RA	55	8
RV	75	80/8
PA	75	80/50
LA	91	12
LV	91	80/20
Abdom. aorta	85	55/45

a) Give three anatomical abnormalities.

....

....

....

Question 10

A 6 week old baby was born at 32 week gestation after a maternal antepartum haemorrhage. Below are some blood test results:

Hb	8.2 g/dl
MCV	80 fl
MCHC	32 g/dl
Reticulocytes	4%
Blood group O positive	
Indirect Coombs test negative	
Blood film crenated cells, several spherocytes	

a) What is the most likely diagnosis?

....

CASE HISTORY PAPER

(Time available: 55 minutes)

1. Answer **all the questions** based upon the following 5 case histories in the spaces provided.

2. When asked (for example) to list 3 diagnoses or investigations, one line will be provided for each answer. If more than the required number of answers are given, the additional answers will not be scored.

Case History 1

A 13 year old African boy known to have sickle cell disease presents with a 2 day history of intermittent abdominal pain.

He has been admitted on many occasions with acute painful crises and in the last two years has required two exchange transfusions during severe sickle chest syndrome. When last seen in the clinic he was well, Hb 8.1 g/dl and taking regular folic acid and penicillin.

Two days previously, after breakfast he suddenly felt a sharp abdominal pain which made him bend double and later feel nauseated. The pain settled for the rest of the day and he slept well. He was well the following day at school until the afternoon when the pain began again. It was present on admission to hospital and was settling.

On examination he is quite a thin boy, apyrexial and looking comfortable. Sclerae are jaundiced, there is no clubbing or cyanosis. Abdomen is soft and moves with respiration. The liver is just palpable 1 cm below the costal margin. He is tender in the epigastric area and right hypochondrium but there is no guarding. The bowel sounds are normal.

Investigations:
  Hb 8.0 g/dl
  WBC 11.4 x 10^9/l
  Platelets 420 x 10^9/l
  Na 131 mmol/l
  K 4.0 mmol/l

Question 1

a) Give the most likely explanation for his symptoms.

  ....

b) What one investigation would be most helpful?

  ....

✓

Case History 2

A 21 year old pregnant woman is rushed to hospital, in labour. She gives birth, at term, to a baby girl in the ambulance. Mother and child are admitted to the postnatal ward where she begins to breast feed. This is her first baby. At 48 hours the baby is noted to be pale. Mother mentions the passage of dark sticky stools in the nappy. On examination, the baby's pulse is 160, respiratory rate 70, no recession. Stools dark and sticky.

Question 2

a) What two investigations would you perform next?

....

....

b) What would be your immediate treatment?

....

Case History 3

An 11 month old girl presents with a three day history of diarrhoea and vomiting. Over the past 24 hours she has become increasingly lethargic with occasional jerking movements of her lower limbs.

On examination she looked 5-10% dehydrated, drowsy and difficult to rouse. Fontanelle felt full, no neck stiffness, apyrexial, no rash, no lymphadenopathy.

Neurological examination revealed increased tone and brisk reflexes in her lower limbs, plantars equivocal. Fundi normal.

Investigations:
    CSF: RBC 50/mm^3
            WBC 3/mm^3 lymphocytes
            no organisms seen
            protein 0.78 g/l
            glucose 2.2 mmol/l

Question 3

a) Give one further investigation that will help to make a diagnosis.

    ....

b) Give two differential diagnoses.

    ....

    ....

Case History 4

A 6 year old girl presents with left lower lobe pneumonia. This responds well to intravenous antibiotics and she is discharged after six days. In her first six years of life she had four episodes of pneumonia, one also in the left lower lobe and the others at different sites. Her first episode was at eighteen months. Between episodes she is active and thriving.

She was born at 39 weeks' gestation and spent twelve hours on the S.C.B.U. with unexplained tachypnoea. This settled, a septic screen was negative and she was returned to her mother.

At three years of age community screening revealed a hearing loss which was due to bilateral serous otitis media. Grommets were inserted.

Question 4

a) What three investigations would you perform?

....

....

....

b) What is the most likely diagnosis?

....

Case History 5

A 13 week old infant is admitted from the child health clinic because of concern over rapid increase in head size. He had been born by forceps delivery at 42 weeks' gestation. There had been some meconium at delivery but the Apgar scores recorded were 7 at 1 minute and 9 at 5 minutes. So far he has been fully immunised and is being bottle fed.

The head size was noted to be above the 97th centile and there were retinal haemorrhages in both fundi. Four small red marks were noticed on the anterior aspect of the chest.

Question 5

a) What is the most likely cause for the increase in head size?

....

b) What three investigations would you perform next?

....

....

....

c) What is your next management step?

....

EXAM 5

DATA INTERPRETATION PAPER

(Time available: 45 minutes)

1. Answer **all 10 of the following questions** in the spaces provided.

2. When asked (for example) to list 3 diagnoses or investigations, one line will be provided for each answer. If more than the required number of answers are given, the additional answers will not be scored.

Question 1

A 5 week old baby presents with a history of vomiting since birth and poor weight gain. On examination he is floppy and lethargic but no other abnormalities are evident.

Investigations
   Na 130 mmol/l
   K 2.0 mmol/l
   Cl 73 mmol/l
   HCO_3 50 mmol/l
   Abdominal ultrasound normal

a) What biochemical abnormality is present?

   ....

b) What investigation should be performed?

   ....

c) What is the most likely diagnosis?

   ....

Question 2

This is the family tree of two families with sensorineural deafness.

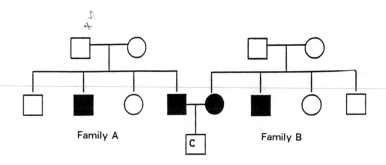

a) What is the inheritance pattern in family A?

....

b) What is the inheritance pattern in family B?

....

c) What is the chance of the offspring indicated having normal hearing?

....

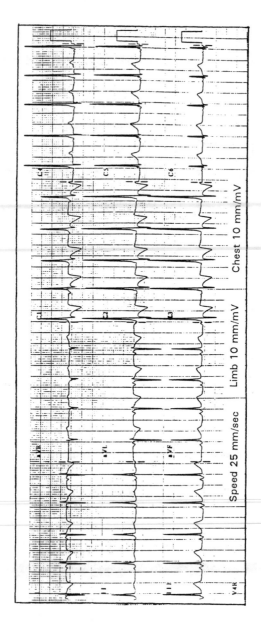

ECG relating to question 3

Question 3

With regard to the ECG shown opposite:

a) What two abnormalities are shown?

....

b) What clinical importance do they have?

....

Question 4

A girl with polyuria has the following serum electrolytes:

Na 145 mmol/l
K 2.8 mmol/l
Cl 95 mmol/l
HCO_3 34 mmol/l
Glucose 6.8 mmol/l

a) Give three possible diagnoses.

....

....

....

Question 5

A 4 year old boy presents with developmental delay. He has mild microcephaly and short palpebral fissures. On cardiovascular examination a soft ejection systolic murmur is heard maximal at the left sternal edge radiating to the carotids.

Biochemistry:

Ca 2.9 mmol/l
PO_4 1.7 mmol/l
Alkaline Phosphatase 113 U/l

a) What is the likely diagnosis?

....

b) What is the cause of the murmur?

....

Question 6

A child can copy the top row of shapes but not the bottom.

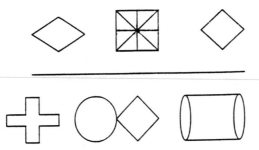

a) How old is he?

....

b) Would you expect him to be able to write his full name?

....

Question 7

The following cardiac catheter data were obtained from a 2 day old infant.

Site	O$_2$ Saturation(%)	Pressure (mmHg)
SVC	63	
IVC	62	
RA	62	mean 4
RV	62	96/5
PA	61	24/5
PV	95	mean 4
LA	80	mean 4
LV	83	90/4
Femoral art.	83	90/55

a) What is the diagnosis?

   ....

b) What immediate treatment should be given?

   ....

c) What is the further management?

   ....

Question 8

A term baby becomes jaundiced at 30 hours of age. The pregnancy and delivery had been uncomplicated.

Total bilirubin 170 μmol/l
Direct bilirubin 10 μmol/l
Hb 15.2 g/dl
WBC 12.1 x 10^9/l
Reticulocytes 5%
Film occasional spherocytes
Blood group A Rh positive
Maternal blood group O Rh negative
Indirect Coombs test positive
Red cell osmotic fragility normal

a) What is the most likely diagnosis?

....

b) Give one further investigation.

....

Question 9

A 2 year old boy was seen with a persistent cough. Examination shows him to be on the 10th centile for weight and height.

Investigations:
Hb 12.0 g/dl
WBC 44 x 10^9/l, 60% lymphocytes, 23% PMN
Platelets 400 x 10^9/l

Chest X-ray patchy opacification right lower lobe

a) What is the diagnosis?

....

Question 10

A 4 day old baby was looking dusky on the post-natal ward. The following were the blood gas results:

	Air	*90% oxygen for 10 minutes*
PaO_2, kPa	6.95	18.6
$PaCO_2$, kPa	4.67	5.01

a) What does this result suggest about the cause of cyanosis?

....

....

....

....

EXAM 6

CASE HISTORY PAPER

(Time available: 55 minutes)

1. Answer **all the questions** based upon the following 5 case histories in the spaces provided.

2. When asked (for example) to list 3 diagnoses or investigations, one line will be provided for each answer. If more than the required number of answers are given, the additional answers will not be scored.

Case History 1

You are asked to see a 15 year old girl in paediatric outpatients. The previous day she had attended casualty following a generalised convulsion with loss of consciousness that lasted about three minutes. She had been at an all night 'rave' party the previous night, arriving home at 4am. She denied taking drugs or alcohol. In casualty she was apyrexial, alert and orientated and had no abnormal neurological signs.

She had one similar convulsion a month ago, which was attributed to alcohol consumption and a very late night. Her parents describe her as 'not a morning person'. She would be unsteady on getting out of bed, and always dropping things until she had properly woken up. The girl felt her clumsiness in the morning was getting worse. Physical and neurological examinations were again entirely normal.

Question 1

a)   What is the most likely diagnosis?

. . . .

b)   What would be the most useful investigation?

. . . .

c)   What would be your next step in her management?

. . . .

Case History 2

A male infant was born by normal vaginal delivery at term to a 29 year old woman, following a normal pregnancy. Apart from a viral illness a month before delivery, the pregnancy was normal. Her membranes ruptured 28 hours before delivery.

The liquor was initially clear, but at delivery meconium was suctioned from the oropharynx by the midwife. The baby was pale, floppy and apnoeic and required ventilation and full intensive therapy.

Laboratory data:
FbC
Hb 11.7 g/dl
WBC $1.4 \times 10^9/l$
Neutrophils 0.3
Platelets 88

Electrolytes
Na 130
K 4.6
U 8
Cr 80
Blood glucose 4

Coagulation
INR 2.7
APTT 48
FDP > 300

Question 2

a)   What is the most likely diagnosis?

. . . .

b)   Give one differential diagnosis.

. . . .

c)   List three antenatal risk factors for the baby's illness.

....

....

....

d)   What is the most important treatment?

....

Case History 3

A 2 month old baby girl has a two month history of vomiting and bloody diarrhoea. She was born at term following a normal pregnancy. She was breast-fed for 2 weeks and then commenced on a cows' milk infant formula. At one month of age her mother reported that she was 'colicky' and very difficult to settle. She developed eczema over her face and flexor surfaces at 6 weeks of age.

The mother is an 18 year old single college student. She lives in a council run hostel for single mothers, and has no contact with her family or the baby's father. Another baby in the hostel has had diarrhoea and vomiting for a few days, but is now better.

The health visitor was extremely concerned as the baby was failing to thrive, and the symptoms persisted.

A stool culture was negative for bacteria and viruses.

The vomiting settled spontaneously after a month. However, she remained irritable and continued to have diarrhoea. Her health visitor changed her milk to a soya based formula. This however had no effect on the diarrhoea.

Question 3

a)   What is the diagnosis?

. . . .

b)   Which procedure would help make the diagnosis?

. . . .

c)   Which immunological tests would help confirm the diagnosis?

. . . .

Case History 4

A 3 year old girl presents with a 6 month history of tiredness and irritability. Her mother reports that she has had a limp for the past 3 months. The parents are both full-time executives and the girl is looked after during the day by a nanny.

The family visited relatives in the USA six months ago. The rest of the families are well.

When examined, the girl was apyrexial and her right knee was swollen and tender. There was a fixed flexion deformity of 20 degrees.

Investigations:
> Hb 9.9 g/dl
> WBC 13
> Plt 410
> ESR 50 mm/hr
> Rheumatoid factor negative

Question 4

a)   What is the diagnosis?

. . . .

b)   What investigation is of prognostic significance?

. . . .

c)   Which further specialised examination is necessary?

. . . .

Case History 5

A 6 year old boy is brought to the Accident and Emergency Department with a sudden onset of swelling of the eyelids and lips, together with hoarseness, wheezing and diarrhoea. Two days previously he had developed a flu-like illness. His parents mentioned that he'd had a milder, similar episode some years previously, but had since been well apart from spells of recurrent abdominal pain. He had been investigated for this but no cause was found. It is the first week of term at a new school.

His mother and grandfather both give a history of having periodic bouts of facial swelling, wheezing and abdominal pain in the past.

Question 5

a)   What is the likely diagnosis?

. . . .

b)   What investigation will confirm the diagnosis?

. . . .

c)   What is the treatment in life-threatening cases?

. . . .

EXAM 6

DATA INTERPRETATION PAPER

(Time available: 45 minutes)

1. Answer **all 10 of the following questions** in the spaces provided.

2. When asked (for example) to list 3 diagnoses or investigations, one line will be provided for each answer. If more than the required number of answers are given, the additional answers will not be scored.

Question 1

A term male infant is born by normal delivery and is well until 6 hours of age. He is noted by a midwife to be cyanosed, pale and apnoeic. Examination reveals micrognathia and a cleft palate.

Blood gas in air
  pH 7.29
  $PaCO_2$ 11
  PaO_2 8.5
  BE -1
  HCO_3 23

a) What emergency management is necessary?

    . . . .

b) What is the likely diagnosis?

    . . . .

Question 2

A 13 year old girl with IDDM is seen because of concern over her poor control of her blood sugars.

She was diagnosed with IDDM one year previously following a history of polyuria and polydipsia. She was initially treated with 4 units of insulin per day by insulin pen injection. Her insulin requirement is now up to 60 units per day and has recently been changed to 4 times a day. There is scanty documentation of blood sugars in her home diary but they are all within the normal range. She says she has never experienced hypoglycaemic episodes at any time of day. She is the middle child in the family.

When seen on this occasion she appeared tall and thin but was otherwise well. Her pubertal development was Tanner Stage 2 with no signs of menarche yet. Examination of her injection sites did not reveal tissue lipotrophy. Her blood results were as follows:

```
HbA1C  12.8%
FBC  Hb  12
     WCC  8
     plt  290
U  6
Na  140
K  3.9
Cr  63
Gluc  6.5
```

a)   What is the cause of her recent poor control?

. . . .

Question 3

14 year old boy complaining of shortness of breath and problems concentrating has the following blood results:

Hb 10.1
MCV 56
RCC 5.5
Serum iron – elevated
Serum ferritin raised
Hb Electrophoresis normal

a) What tests would aid the diagnosis?

. . . .

b) What is the most likely diagnosis?

. . . .

Question 4

A 2 week old boy presents with a short history of vomiting and collapse. He has the following blood results:

Arterial blood gas   pH 7.32
                      pCO$_2$ 5.9
                      pO$_2$ 9.8
                      bicarbonate 19
Na 125
K 5.8
gluc 4.9

a) What is the most important diagnostic test?

. . . .

b) What is the most likely diagnosis?

. . . .

Question 5

A baby born at 28 weeks gestation is now 100 days old and has chronic lung disease, requiring nasal cannula oxygen. He develops a cough and respiratory distress, with an increasing oxygen requirement. RSV bronchiolitis is diagnosed. An arterial blood gas shows:

pH 7.2
pCO_2 13
pO_2 11.2
bic 28
base excess +6

a)   How would you classify his acid-base status?

. . . .

b)   What would you do next?

. . . .

Question 6

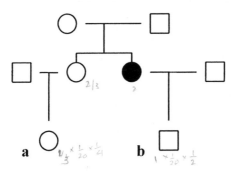

The diagram above is a pedigree of a family where the shaded circle represents the proband with cystic fibrosis.

a)   Assuming the population carrier rate is 1 in 20 what is the probability of each of the offspring (**a** and **b**) following having CF?

. . . .

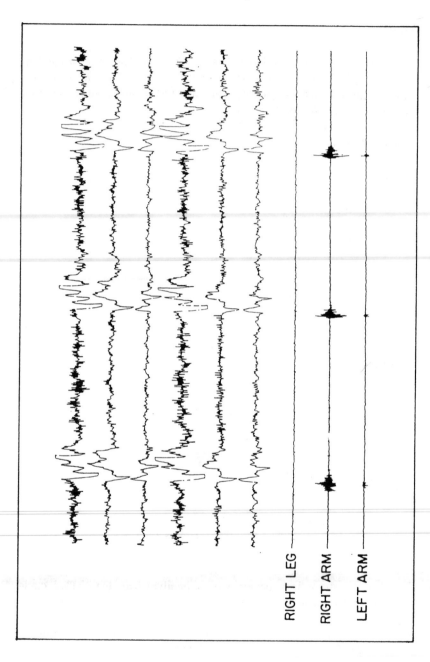

EMG/EEG relating to question 7

Question 7

A previously bright 9 year old girl, recently arrived in the UK from Boston, USA, is noted by her teachers to be falling behind academically. Her mother reports that she frequently drops her knife and fork and has recently noticed intermittent jerking of her arms and legs.

See EMG/EEG shown opposite

a)   What is the diagnosis?

. . . .

b)   How can this be confirmed?

. . . .

Question 8

A 1 year old boy is seen in casualty because of excessive crying. His mother reports that he is not satisfied with additional milk, but is settled with water. His father was treated for pulmonary TB 8 months ago.

Results are as follows:

Na 158 mmol/l
K 4.0 mmol/l
Urea 4.1 mmol/l
Creatinine 58 mmol/l
Glucose 5.0 mmol/l
Serum osmolality 340 mOsmol/l
Urine osmolality 80 mOsmol/l

a)   What is the diagnosis?

. . . .

b)   What is the likely underlying cause?

. . . .

c)   What is the treatment?

. . . .

Question 9

A 5 year old girl presented with a 6 month history of irritability, lethargy and low grade fevers. Her gait became waddling and her mother pointed out that she had difficulty in climbing stairs. She developed a pink-purple rash over her face, eye-lids and limbs.

Investigations:
   Hb 10
   ESR 22
   CRP < 5
   CK 380
   ANA positive
   Rheumatoid factor negative
   Antinuclear antibody negative

a)   What is the diagnosis?

   . . . .

b)   Name two confirmatory diagnostic tests.

   . . . .

   . . . .

c)   What is the treatment?

   . . . .

Question 10

A 15 year old boy is referred by his GP following a year long history of generalised malaise and weight loss. His height and weight have both fallen to the third centile and on examination his testicular volume is 6 mls and he has sparse pubic hair and no axillary hair. He is noted to be pale but the rest of the examination is unremarkable.

Investigations:
   Fbc Hb 9.8 g/dl
   MCV 65
   WCC 13
   Plt 685
   Ferritin 11
   ESR 9
   CRP 40
   Albumin 29

a)   What is the likely diagnosis?

   . . . .

b)   How would you confirm this diagnosis?

   . . . .

c)   What treatment is effective?

   . . . .

EXAM 7

CASE HISTORY PAPER

(Time available: 55 minutes)

1. Answer **all the questions** based upon the following 5 case histories in the spaces provided.

2. When asked (for example) to list 3 diagnoses or investigations, one line will be provided for each answer. If more than the required number of answers are given, the additional answers will not be scored.

Case History 1

An 11 year old boy presents with poor school performance recently exacerbated by frequent bullying. On examination he was tall (> 97 centile) with a pectus carinatum chest deformity and mild scoliosis. He wears glasses to correct a severe myopia and with these on his visual acuity was normal. Facially, he resembled his father with a noticeably small jaw and downsloping palpebral fissures. His chest was clear on examination but he had a pansystolic murmur grade 4/6. He was normotensive and examination of central nervous system was normal.

Question 1

a) What is the most likely diagnosis?

    . . . .

b) What investigations would you do next?

    . . . .

c) What is the likely cause of the heart murmur?

    . . . .

Case History 2

A 13 year old girl presented with a 2 month history of joint pain. She was a keen gymnast but had to stop because her knees had become particularly swollen. There was no significant past medical history and on examination she appeared well, with no fever and no rash. Her joints were not swollen but facial and ankle oedema were evident. There were no other abnormalities on examination.

Investigations:
  BP 135/80
  Hb 11.2
  WBC 7.4
  Na 136
  K 5.5
  Urea 6.0
  Creatinine 45 micromol/l
  Albumin 20 g/l
  Protein 44 g/l
  ESR 80 mm/hr
  ASOT normal
  Urine WBC 35/mm^3 RBC 45/mm^3
  Autoantibody screen anti-nuclear factor positive
  Anti-double stranded DNA 300 IU (normal <50)

Question 2

a)   What is the most likely diagnosis?

   . . . .

b)   What investigations would best confirm your diagnosis?

   . . . .

c)   What would be the treatment of choice?

   . . . .

Case History 3

A 2 month old baby boy is brought to the Accident and Emergency Department by his mother with a month long history of intermittent abdominal distension. He was born by normal delivery and passed meconium within 24 hours. He was solely breast-fed until 3 weeks, when cows' formula milk was introduced as a supplement. At first he opened his bowels 5 or 6 times per day, but by 4 weeks this was only every 5 to 6 days. His mother withdrew the formula milk at 5 weeks, but the bowel pattern remained the same. Prune juice had no effect. His mother describes the baby straining during passage of hard pellet-like stools. There was no blood passed with the stool.

His mother found that by giving glycerine suppositories obtained over the counter, the baby passed a large amount of wind and there was a gush of a large amount of soft stool.

Question 3

a) What important investigation should be ordered urgently?

. . . .

b) Which condition needs to be excluded and how is this done?

. . . .

c) What important complication needs to be watched for?

. . . .

Case History 4

A 14 year old boy is admitted to hospital following a generalised tonic clonic convulsion. He had been complaining of mild frontal headaches for the past two weeks. They were not associated with visual disturbance or vomiting, and were relieved by paracetamol. Upon coming home from school that afternoon, he had complained of a severe and sudden onset headache. His mother gave him paracetamol, but 5 minutes later she noticed that he began convulsing, with shaking of both arms and legs. His mother described him as healthy, but she had found him sniffing glue when he was aged 12. He had subsequently stopped doing this. According to his mother he was an above average student and there had not been any recent change in his school progress.

By the time he had arrived in the Emergency Department, he had been convulsing for 30 minutes. He was drowsy and responsive only to painful stimuli. His temperature was 37.6 °C, pulse 54, BP 160/90. His pupils were equal and sluggishly reactive to light. The optics discs margins appeared slightly blurred.

Question 4

a)   After stabilising his general condition, what two actions should you take?

. . . .

. . . .

b)   What is the most likely diagnosis?

. . . .

Case History 5

A term male infant was born by normal delivery to a mother with insulin dependent diabetes. His birth weight was 4.5 kg. He was noted not to move his right arm and the right radial and brachial pulses were not palpable. He was pink at delivery.

Laboratory data:
Hb 21
PCV 70
Plt 280
WCC 14.3
Neutrophils 9
Na 139
K 4.2
U 6
Cr 80
Blood glucose 2.1

Question 5

a) Name two urgent interventions.

....

....

b) Name two radiological investigations, which can be performed on the neonatal unit in order to assess the baby's arm?

....

....

c) Name two recognised congenital abnormalities seen in infants of diabetic mothers.

....

....

d) Name two possible causes of right arm paresis.

....

....

EXAM 7

DATA INTERPRETATION PAPER

(Time available: 45 minutes)

1. Answer **all 10 of the following questions** in the spaces provided.

2. When asked (for example) to list 3 diagnoses or investigations, one line will be provided for each answer. If more than the required number of answers are given, the additional answers will not be scored.

Question 1

A 29 week gestation baby boy who is 2 weeks old remains on a ventilator. He continues to receive TPN. The neonatal nurses note a temperature instability. Lab investigations show:

Hb 12.9 g/dl
WCC 20×10^9/l
Plt 99×10^9/l
ABG pH 7.28
pCO_2 5.0
pO_2 9.8
Bic 17
BE -6
Blood glucose 10.0
INR 1.3
APTT 40 seconds
CRP 30

a)   What investigations would you perform?

. . . .

b)   What is the likely cause?

. . . .

c)   What further action would you consider in view of your above answer?

. . . .

Question 2

A 5 day old term baby has right-sided seizures. The results of investigations are as follows:

Hb 11 g/l
WCC 6.4x10^9/l
Urea 5.2 mmol/l
Na 139 mmol/l
K 4.4 mmol/l
Ca 2.1 mmol/l
Gluc 4 mmol/l
ABG normal

a)   Name three further investigations.

. . . .

. . . .

. . . .

Question 3

A 10 year old girl presented with an intracranial tumour at the age of 9. She was treated with cranial radiotherapy. She subsequently failed to grow.

Investigations:

Thyroxine 58 nmol/l

Insulin tolerance test

Time (mins)	0	20	30	60	90	120
Glucose (mmol/l)	4	2	2	4.2	7.1	8.0
Cortisol (nmol/l)	20	50	80	85	78	68
Growth Hormone (mU/l)	< 0.5	0.6	0.6	< 0.5	< 0.5	< 0.5
TSH (mU/l)	3.1	14		30		
Prolactin (mU/l)	699	1350		1010		

a) From the above data, give three endocrine abnormalities.

....

....

....

b) What is the treatment for each of these?

....

....

....

Question 4

A short 2 year old boy has a long history of steatorrhoea and recurrent chest and skin infections.

Laboratory results:
  Hb 10.1
  WCC 3.5
  Neutrophils 0.6
  Platelets 90
  Faecal elastase 150 (normal > 500)
  Sweat test sodium 21 mmol/l
        chloride 23 mmol/l
  Femoral head X-rays metaphyseal dysplasia

a) What is the diagnosis?

. . . .

b) What medication may reduce the diarrhoea?

. . . .

c) What bowel side-effect is associated with this medication?

. . . .

Question 5

A 10 kg, 14 month old girl has vomiting and diarrhoea for a day. She is irritable and has a capillary refill time of 3 seconds. Skin turgor has a 'doughy' feel. She is felt to be 7.5% dehydrated.

Data:

Sodium	160 mmol/l ↑
Potassium	4.0 mmol/l
Urea	12.1 mmol/l
Creatinine	140 mmol/l

a)   What is the diagnosis?

....

b)   What is this child's fluid deficit and maintenance requirements?

....

c)   What type of fluid would you use initially?

....

Question 6

EEG

Overleaf is the EEG from a 7 month old boy.

a)   What is this appearance called?

....

b)   What is the diagnosis?

....

c)   What is the treatment?

....

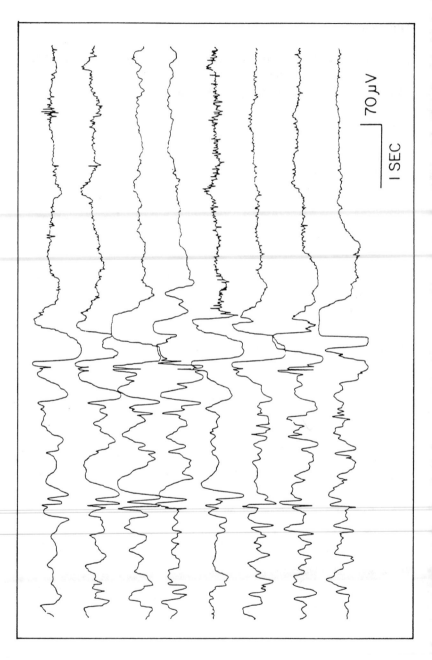

70 μV

I SEC

EEG relating to question 6

Question 7

A 13 year old boy from Ireland is referred with a history of recurrent jaundice. Liver function test results are as follows:

Total bili 60 µmol/l
Conjug bili 3 µmol/l
Tot prot 66 g/l
ALT 13 iu/l
ALP 120 iu/l
Haptoglobin 0.1 g/l (0.3–2 g/l)
Hb 9.0 g/dl
WCC 8.4x10⁹/l
Plt 325x10⁹/l

a)   What is the diagnosis?

. . . .

b)   How can this be confirmed?

. . . .

Question 8

A 3 year old boy presents with developmental delay. His vision and hearing have been tested and are normal. He has had no fits or other illnesses. Although his gross and fine motor milestones were achieved within the normal ranges, he only has one recognisable word and little babble. Formal developmental testing confirms marked delays in his verbal and performance skills. He has a 1 year old sister who already seems to have more speech than he does. There is no significant family history. On examination he is normally grown, head circumference is on the 50th centile, there are no neurocutaneous lesions, no obvious dysmorphic features and neurological examination is normal.

a)   What three investigations would be the most useful in this case?

. . . .

. . . .

. . . .

Question 9

A 5 month old girl with severe weeping eczema has been managed for 3 weeks with topical steroid wraps. The child in the next door cubicle has returned the day before from paediatric intensive care where he was treated for meningococcal septicaemia. The eczema had improved and the steroid wraps were stopped. On the day prior to discharge, she began vomiting. On examination her fontanelle felt full, she had bilateral papilloedema but she was alert and had no focal neurological signs. There was no evidence of a rash. Cardiovascular system was stable.

a)   What is the diagnosis?

. . . .

b)   What investigation should be performed initially?

. . . .

c)   How should this baby be treated?

. . . .

Question 10

A 4 year old boy is rushed to casualty after having a febrile convulsion. The paramedics gave him a single dose of 5 mg rectal diazepam and the seizure stopped after 5 minutes. On arrival his arterial blood gas whilst receiving face mask oxygen is:

pH 7.19
pO_2 9.1
pCO_2 12.2
Bicarbonate 21
Base deficit -3

a)   What abnormality is seen on this blood gas and what is its most likely cause?

. . . .

b)   What diameter/size endotracheal tube would you use if intubation was required?

. . . .

ANSWERS AND TEACHING NOTES

EXAM 1 : CASE HISTORIES

Case History 1

a) Colonoscopy and biopsy
b) Crohn's Disease

Discussion

Crohn's disease has recently increased in incidence to about 5 per 100,000, equal to ulcerative colitis.

Whilst classical presentations are well known, several more unusual presentations are described. Anorexia nervosa is characteristically associated with an abnormal body image which is unlikely in Crohn's disease.

As it affects the entire GI tract, cheilitis is important to note as is the characteristic full upper lip of aphthous ulceration. The diagnosis has even been made following upper GI endoscopy revealing aphthous ulceration in the oesophagus.

In diagnosis, ESR or more specifically C-reactive protein may be raised; barium meal and follow through would also be an unacceptable answer.

References
Walker-Smith JA, *Clinical and Diagnostic features of Chronic Inflammatory Bowel Disease in Childhood*, Chronic inflammatory bowel disease in childhood. Balliere's Clin Gastroenterolgy 1994;**8**:65-82
Hyams JS, *Crohn's disease in children*, Pediatric Clinics of North America. 43(1):255-77, 1996 Feb

Case History 2

a)   Organic and amino acid screen
b)   Inborn error of metabolism

Key Points
- Early presentation
- Vomiting after milk feeds
- Severe metabolic acidosis
- The CSF results are normal for a neonate
- Prematurity is not relevant to the answer
- The cerebral ultrasound appearance is of non-specific cerebral oedema reflecting the effect of acidosis
- No more specific wording than inborn error of metabolism is requires as the final answer

Discussion

Although the range of possible symptoms in babies with metabolic errors is wide, two frequent patterns exist. The first begins with vomiting, acidosis and circulatory disturbance, followed by depressed consciousness and convulsions. This is suggestive of the organic acidaemias.

The second pattern is dominated by neurological features with lethargy, refusal to feed, drowsiness, unconsciousness and convulsions. Hypotonia may be a marked feature. Primary defects of the urea cycle and disorders such as glycine encephalopathy and β-alaninaemia should then be considered.

Answers mentioning sepsis and blood cultures would also score some marks. Alternative investigations are blood glucose, calcium and drug screen.

Reference
Hoffman GF, *Selective screening for inborn errors of metabolism,* European Journal of Pediatrics. 153 (7 suppl 1):52–8, 1994.

Case History 3

a) Paired acute and convalescent serum titres for mycoplasma
   Blood cultures
   Immunofluorescent staining of the sputum
b) Oral erythromycin

Key Points

- Dry cough
- Systematic illness
- Headaches
- An important clue is that the illness has not responded to first line antibiotics

Discussion

This is a typical history for an atypical pneumonia. Note also the anaemia and reticulocytosis suggesting cold agglutinins directed against red cells. The budgerigar (but not the cat) would be a relevant vector for *Chlamydia psittaci*. Note that whilst *Mycoplasma pneumoniae* may produce any X-ray appearance including lobar consolidation, *C. psittaci* generally produces bilateral patchy consolidation. Blood cultures are positive in less than 25% of community acquired pneumonias. Antibody titres are the main diagnostic tests available for atypical pneumonias. Mycoplasma specific IgM is a useful early test but not widely available.

Case History 4

a)   Inhalation of foreign body with supervening chest infection
b)   Bronchoscopy

Key Points
- The blow to the chest is irrelevant
- 'Sudden paroxysm of severe coughing' should be enough to raise the possibility of inhalation of a foreign body

Discussion

Edible nuts make up 50% of intrabronchial foreign bodies. 66% are diagnosed in the first week, others may go unrecognised for months. Most lodge in a main or stem bronchus, right side more often than left. If the clinical and radiological pattern of illness is suggestive, bronchoscopy should be carried out even without history of inhalation.

Delayed diagnosis may present as
      recurrent wheeze
      persistent chest infection
      chronic cough with haemoptysis
      lung collapse with respiratory failure

Late diagnosis may result in infection distal to the bronchial obstruction. Removal may fail if the foreign body breaks up. On occasion, if removal fails, thoracotomy and resection may be required. Follow up after successful removal should be by the ventilation perfusion lung scan, a more sensitive index of lung damage than chest X-ray in this case. Ventilation-perfusion scan will show a persistent abnormality if the foreign body has been in situ for more than 24 hours.

Case History 5

a) Full blood count and film
b) Blood pressure and weight
c) Haemolytic uraemic syndrome

Key points
- Haemolytic uraemic syndrome (H.U.S.) now affects 150 children a year in the UK and should be considered in any preschool child with bloody diarrhoea
- Pallor and jaundice in this case reflect haemolysis
- A blood film will demonstrate anaemia, thrombocytopenia and features of microangiopathic haemolytic anaemia

Discussion

H.U.S. defines a group of conditions in which microangiopathic haemolytic anaemia coexists with acute renal impairment. It now represents the most common cause of childhood acute renal failure in Europe. Abdominal pain is not uncommon and appendicitis or intussusception may be suspected.

Stool cultures may yield *Escherichia coli* serotype 0157:H7 producing verotoxin. The D+ form with prodromal diarrhoea has a good long term outcome in 80% of cases if dialysis is avoided. The less common D-form, which may be familial or relapsing, carries a poor prognosis.

Reference
Neuhaus TJ, Calonder S, Leumann EP, *Heterogeneity of atypical haemolytic uraemic syndromes,* Archives of Disease in Childhood. 76(6):518-21, 1997 Jun.

EXAM 1 : DATA INTERPRETATIONS

Question 1

a)   Sickle cell beta + thalassaemia
b)   Beta + thalassaemia

Discussion

Haemoglobin	*Structure*	*Comment*
A	α2β2	92% of all adult Hb
A2	α2δ2	2% of adult Hb elevated in β thal
F	α2γ2	normal haemoglobin in fetus stays elevated in β thal
Barts	β4	Found in α thal. Biologically useless
H	γ4	100% of haemoglobin in homozygous α thal, biologically useless

Electrophoresis

Sickle cell disease	HbS, no HbA HbF variable 5-15%
Sickle trait	HbS 25-45% HbA
β - Thal trait	HbA HbA2 > 3.5% makes the diagnosis ± HbF
β - Thal major	HbA virtually absent HbF majority HbA2 variable low/normal/raised
Sickle thalassaemia	HbS HbF ± HbA

Clinical and haematological manifestations of sickle thalassaemia are variable, much of this due to two types of abnormal beta chain synthesis.

β° denotes no beta chain production. β^+ small amounts beta chain synthesis. Patients with sickle cell thalassaemia in general do not require blood transfusions, but many suffer severe sickle-cell crises.

Question 2

a)   X linked hypophosphataemic rickets

Type	Ca	PO$_4$	AKP	PTH	25(OH)D3	1.25(OH)D3	AA-uria
D defct	↓/N	↓/N	↑	↑	↓	↓/N	+
D dep 1	↓	↓/N	↑↑	↑	N	↓↓	+ +
D dep 2	↓	↓/N	↑↑	↑	N	↑↑	+
X linked	N	↓↓	↑	N	N	N/↓	-

D defct = Vitamin D deficient
D dep 1 = Vitamin D dependent type 1
D dep 2 = Vitamin D dependent type 2
X linked = Familial, X-linked hypophosphataemic rickets

Question 3

a)   X-linked dominant.
This is a better answer than simple autosomal dominant.
Note absence of transmission from male to male.

Question 4

a)   A normal EEG

Discussion

EEGs are common data questions. They are not complicated and simply a matter of pattern recognition. You will need to know about seven 'patterns' as well as the normal trace. Here is a simple guide:

1.   Read the question, noting the age and drug treatment.

2.   Check the time marker. This is usually at the top of the EEG in 1 second intervals and allows calculation of the frequency of any complex.

3.   Check the amplitude scale.

4.   Check the montage (map). This is basically a pictorial representation of the sites between which a potential difference is being measured.

5.   Now look at the traces:
    What is its nature – spike/sharp wave, slow wave, complex
    Is it present in all channels (generalised)
    Is it in one area only (focal)

6.   Is there a pattern?
    3 per second spike wave in absences
    Periodic complexes – SSPE/Herpes simplex encephalitis
    Chaotic large voltage complex – Hypsarrhythmia
    Rolandic spikes etc.

Normal EEGs

In young or premature babies there is little difference between the sleeping and waking state. Electrical activity is irregular and intermittent so interpretation requires a great deal of skill. With increasing maturity the cerebral potentials become rhythmic and a dominant rhythm emerges, initially slow 4 to 6 Hz becoming faster to form the alpha rhythm 8 to 12 Hz characteristic of the adult EEG. This EEG shows 8 to 12 Hz characteristic of the adult EEG. This EEG shows 8 to 12 alpha waves, amplitudes less than 50 μV.

Question 5

a) Cystic fibrosis
b) Hyponatraemia, hypokalaemic metabolic alkalosis
c) Pseudo-Bartter's syndrome secondary to hyperaldosteronism in cystic fibrosis.

Discussion

Sweat test
a) 100 mg of sweat is the minimum that should be collected for a test to be valid.
b) Normal children aged between 4 weeks and 13 years have Na < 60 mmol and Cl < 15 mmol/l.
c) The test is consistent with cystic fibrosis if Na > 60 and Cl > 70 mmol/l.

The electrode pattern is termed pseudo-Bartter's, producing the same hypokalaemic alkalosis as seen in Bartter's syndrome, with hyperplasia of the juxtaglomerular apparatus. There is persistent hyponatraemia and hypo-kalaemia secondary to excessive sweat electrode loss. These children need large quantities of supplemental sodium and potassium during the first few months of life.

Question 6

a) Restrictive
b) Myasthenia gravis
   Fibrosing alveolitis
   Scoliosis

Discussion

Forced vital capacity is the total volume of gas expelled during forced expiration. This volume is reduced in conditions with reduced pulmonary compliance (stiff lungs), reduced lung volume or neuromuscular disease. The volume of this gas expired within the first second is the FEV_1. This is also reduced in restrictive lung disease but proportionately to the total lung volume. As a result, FEV_1/FVC is normal in restrictive lung disease.

Question 7

a)   1½ years

Question 8

a)   Ventricular septal defect
     Right ventricular outflow tract obstruction
b)   Fallot's tetralogy

Cardiac catheter data are best interpreted by following saturation and then pressure measurements through each chamber in anatomical sequence from systematic venous to systematic arterial. It may be simpler to draw a diagram listing the abnormalities (see normal values).

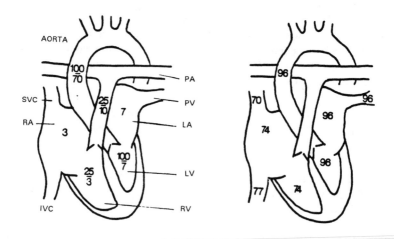

normal pressure measurements (mmHg)   normal oxygen saturation (%)

There is a step-up in oxygen saturation between right atrium and right ventricle implying a left to right shunt at ventricular level.

The pressure gradient between the right ventricle and pulmonary artery implies right ventricular outflow tract obstruction.

These features, in addition to desaturation seen in the aorta suggest the diagnosis of Fallot's tetralogy.

Question 9

a) Conductive hearing loss
b) Serous otitis media

Discussion

Measurement of the thresholds for air and bone conduction are usually obtained by pure tone audiometry. Stimuli of different frequencies ranging from 250 to 8,000 Hz are emitted at different intensities above the threshold of normal hearing.

Key Points

- A sound made through a headphone of a standard audiometer will also be heard in the contralateral ear if the source in that ear is 50dB or greater. At this stage, masking of the non-test ear has to be undertaken.

- For bone conduction testing when the vibrator is placed on the skull, there is virtually no loss of sound heard in the non-test ear, thus masking should always be undertaken.

In this example there is a wide threshold between air conduction and bone conduction, an 'air-bone gap'. This implies the hearing loss is due to a malfunction of the conducting system of the external and middle ear, rather than a sensori-neural mechanism.

Conductive deafness is the most common type of hearing loss in children. It may be due to secretory otitis media, acute otitis media or congenital abnormalities of the external or middle ear.

Intermittent conductive deafness, provided speech and language are not delayed, is reviewed with audiograms and tympanometry and may resolve spontaneously.

Persistent hearing loss due to middle ear fluid is an indication for referral to an ENT surgeon for possible myringotomy/grommets or adenoidectomy.

Question 10

a)   Septic screen including lumbar puncture
b)   Congenital adrenal hypoplasia
c)   Salt, hydrocortisone and fludrocortisone

This is a sick male infant who on admission has lost more than 10% of his bodyweight and is passing a dilute urine with inappropriately high sodium content. Obviously sepsis needs to be excluded and overwhelming urinary tract infection mimics this picture.

Congenital adrenal hyperplasia should be the working clinical diagnosis once sepsis is ruled out. However, the results show that 17-hydroxyprogesterone is low and distal metabolites are also low (see steroid synthesis pathway). Congenital adrenal hypoplasia is less common than hyperplasia which itself is rare. 21-hydrolase deficiency is the most common variety.

EXAM 2 : CASE HISTORIES

Case History 1

a) Accidental drug ingestion, phenothiazine group
b) Good prognosis if supportive management of airway, breathing and circulation is satisfactory

Key Points
- Oculogyric crises in children are most commonly the result of drug ingestion
- Look for clues in the history such as recent bereavement, schizophrenia, travel sickness etc
- Learn normal values for CSF; note the different ranges for neonates and older children. This result is normal.

Discussion

Overdosage with phenothiazines causes hypotension, hypothermia, cardiac arrythmias, convulsions and extrapyramidal reactions. Treatment is supportive and symptomatic. Dystonic reactions may be treated with benztropine or procyclidine injection. Diazepam may be used to control convulsions.

Case History 2

a)   Pericardial aspiration and biopsy with staining and culture for T.B.
     Echocardiography
b)   Tuberculous constrictive pericarditis

Key Point
   • Asian origin and long history of malaise should alert one to the
     possibility of T.B.

Several vital clinical points
It is unusual not to be able to palpate the apex beat in a thin boy. The JVP is
raised and there is hepatomegaly, ascites (transudate) out of proportion to the
signs and symptoms of heart disease. Mantoux test may be negative in severe
active T.B. It may be positive if 1:1,000 strength is used.

Discussion

Constrictive pericarditis is caused by a wide variety of diseases, most cases
probably originating as pericardial inflammation with effusion. The
pericardium may become thick, fibrous and calcified, impeding cardiac
filling.

Chest X-ray may show a small heart and calcification on lateral views, or be
normal as in this example. ECG characteristically shows low voltage QRS
complexes and T wave inversion. The echocardiogram may demonstrate
thickened pericardium and abnormal motion of the ventricular septum and
posterior left ventricular wall.

Standard antituberculous chemotherapy (rifampicin, isoniazid and
pyrazinamide for 2 months then rifampicin and isoniazid for 4 months). An
eleven week course of prednisolone is advised and surgical removal of a
substantial proportion of the pericardium is required. Pyridoxine should be
taken during antituberculous therapy.

Reference
Strang JI, *Tuberculous pericarditis*, Journal of Infection. 35(3):215-9, 1997
Nov.

Case History 3

a) Renal vein thrombosis
b) Renal ultrasound scan
   Blood culture and sensitivity
   Serum creatinine
c) Hypernatraemia
   Intracranial haemorrhage
   Hypertension

Key Points

- The age group, preceding diarrhoea and palpable kidney make the diagnosis of renal vein thrombosis likely
- Thrombocytopenia and uraemia make this even more likely
- It is reasonable to ask for serum creatinine as this is not given in the question

Discussion

One third of all cases of renal vein thrombosis are detected in the first week of life. Severity varies from grave bilateral involvement to focal involvement of one kidney. Asphyxia, prematurity, dehydration, sepsis and maternal diabetes are possible predisposing factors. In severe cases, peritoneal dialysis and intensive care on a paediatric nephrology unit is indicated. Careful follow up is required as the affected kidney may cause severe hypertension via a renin mediated pathway and should in that case be removed.

Reference
Andrew M, Brooker LA, *Hemostatic complications in renal disorders of the young,* Pediatric Nephrology. 10(1):88-99, 1996 Feb.

Case History 4

a) Severe combined immunodeficiency
b) *Pneumocystis carinii*
c) High dose intravenous co-trimoxazole

Key point
  • Early death in a first degree relative should arouse suspicion of recessively inherited disorders

Discussion

This is a familial immune deficiency with early onset. There is panhypogammaglobulinaemia with low normal white count and absent lymphadenopathy in the presence of diarrhoea and pneumonia. No differential count is given but excluding eosinophils the white count is 3.3.

Agammaglobulinaemia alone presents usually at 4 to 6 months when maternally transferred antibodies are exhausted, diarrhoea also is not a common presenting feature. Thus combined humoral and cellular deficiency exists.

Wiskott-Aldrich is a possibility but usually is associated with thrombocytopenia, increased IgA, normal IgA and half normal IgM levels. SCID has many familial forms in both autosomal and sex linked recessive forms. The skin rash may be chronic candida.

Functional antibodies such as isohaemagglutinins will be absent and there will be absent sensitivity to candida skin testing. Chronic rotavirus carriage is common. Purine nucleoside phosphorylase or adenosine deaminase levels may be diminished in the parents.

Management is supportive until a histocompatible bone marrow donor becomes available. Blood transfusions should be irradiated to reduce the risk of graft versus host reaction.

Case History 5

a) Ketotic hypoglycaemia
b) Carefully controlled provocation fast

Key points
- Note the low birth weight, neuroglycopenic symptoms of ataxia and irritability after overnight fast
- Fasting glucose is well below normal values
- Phenobarbitone has been started for the hypoglycaemic fits and does not necessarily imply that the child has idiopathic epilepsy

Discussion

Ketotic hypoglycaemia is the most common cause of hypoglycaemia and presents usually between 1 and 5 years of age. Affected children (usually boys, M:F 2:1) are small and thin. The basic biochemical defect is unknown but hepatic glycogen is known to be depleted and it is postulated that there is a failure in mobilisation of amino acids from muscle for gluconeogenesis in starvation. Due to accelerated starvation, free fatty acid oxidation is increased giving the disorder its name.

The diagnosis is established by excluding metabolic errors and hormone deficiencies. Either with a carefully supervised provocative fast or prior to a spontaneous episode of hypoglycaemia, urine will become ketotic prior to hypoglycaemia and serial blood glucose should demonstrate impending hypoglycaemia within 8 to 16 hours (24 to 36 in normal children). Simultaneous measurements should be as follows:

Insulin	low
GH	elevated
Cortisol	elevated
Thyroxine	normal
Free fatty acids	elevated
Beta hydroxybutyrate	elevated
Ketones	elevated
Amino acids	decreased alanine
Urine	
Reducing substances	negative

143

| Ketones marked | positive |
| Organic acids | elevated ketones only |

In patients with ketotic hypoglycaemia, there is no response to glucagon in the fasted state but a response is present in the fed state. Glucagon stimulation test should not be necessary if the provocation test is successful.

During a hypoglycaemic attack the child should be given glucose in its most convenient form. Children do well with frequent high protein, high carbohydrate meals (4 or 5 a day). During periods of illness or fasting, high carbohydrate drinks should be offered at frequent intervals. Spontaneous remission occurs by 9 to 10 years.

Reference
Haymond MW, Pagliara AS, *Ketotic hypoglycaemia,* Clinics in Endocrinology & Metabolism, 12(2):447-62, 1983 Jul.

EXAM 2 : DATA INTERPRETATIONS

Question 1

a) Nephrotic syndrome due to minimal change nephritis
b) 24 hour urine protein/creatinine estimation
    Complement levels
    Blood pressure
    Serum (creatinine)
c) Careful fluid management
    Prednisolone 60 mg/m^2 until urine protein free, then 40 mg/m^2 for a
    month
    Penicillin

Minimal change nephritis is the most common pathology underlying childhood nephrotic syndrome. There is an increased incidence amongst the Asian population. Complement level is normal in minimal change but low in more serious renal disease such as SLE, post-streptococcal nephritis, SBE, cryoglobulinaemia and mesangiocapillary glomerulonephritis.

Question 2

a)   Primary generalised non-convulsant epilepsy (Childhood absence)
b)   Hyperventilation
c)   No

Discussion

Childhood absence epilepsy

Clinical characteristics
a)   Age at onset 3-13 years
b)   Normal neurological examination and intelligence
c)   Seizures are typical absences (simple or complex) at onset, followed or
      not by generalised tonic-clonic seizures

EEG features
a)   Background is normal
b)   Ictal shows bilateral, synchronous, symmetrical spike waves, usually at
      3 Hz spontaneously and/or activated by hyperventilation

If these criteria are satisfied further neuroimaging is not necessary prior to
treatment with either ethosuximide or sodium valproate.

Question 3

a)   50% of boys will have a low G6PD
b)   50% of girls will have a marginally low G6PD

The G6PD enzyme is on the X chromosome. G6PD is the rate limiting
enzyme of the pentose phosphate pathway and so important for protecting the
red cell from oxidant stress. More than 100 distinct enzyme variants of G6PD
have been documented.

Question 4

a)   GH deficiency
     Primary hypothyroidism
     GnRH deficiency

Pituitary damage following cranial irradiation is common, GH deficiency occurring in 97% of cases, with peak incidence 2 years after radiotherapy. This boy, having a medulloblastoma, would also have had spinal irradiation, accounting for thyroid damage as reflected in the high TSH levels. This occurs in about 30% of cases. GnRH deficiency is less common.

Question 5

a)   Acquired Immune Deficiency Syndrome (AIDS)
b)   Polymerase chain amplification of HIV nucleic acid
     cd4:cd8 ratio

Discussion

Materno-fetal transmission is responsible for 80% of paediatric HIV infection in the U.K. With routine screening of blood products, the number of children infected through transfusion of blood or products has been minimised.

The vertical transmission risk in Europe is about 13% (i.e. the risk of the child being HIV antibody positive at 18 months); the risk is higher in Africa for various reasons.

Clinical features
Presenting symptoms – 75% are non-specific, including
     failure to thrive
     recurrent bacterial infections
     chronic diarrhoea
     skin infections
there may also be hepatosplenomegaly and lymphadenopathy

Neurodevelopment
     developmental delay
     regression of developmental milestones
     acquired microcephaly
     gait abnormalities

Pulmonary disease
> *Pneumocystis carinii* pneumonia
> lymphoid interstitial pneumonitis

Secondary infection
> recurrent infection of respiratory tract with encapsulated organisms
> (*Pneumocystis, Haemophilus*)
> recurrent meningitis; abscesses

Diagnosis
Before 18 months when HIV antibody may be still passively acquired:
a)   polymerase chain reaction, amplifies extremely small amounts of host nucleic acid to detectable levels. This forms the basis of a very sensitive test which will detect a single molecule of viral nucleic acid amongst the DNA of a host cell.
b)   Polyclonal hypergammaglobulinaemia. This has been shown to be sensitive and specific as early as 3 months.
c)   Low cd4:cd8 ratio. Specific but not as sensitive as hypergammagloulinaemia.
d)   Clinical criteria. In the early stages these are probably the least sensitive and specific.

Treatment
Trials currently underway using AZT and intravenous immunoglobulin therapy. Little information at present about correct doses or frequency of AZT in children. In adults AZT has not been shown to alter the rates of seroconversion.

Question 6

a)   Long PR interval
     Superior axis
     Neonatal RS progression
b)   Atrioventricular septal defect

Question 7

a) Unilateral high voltage centrotemporal spikes
b) Benign childhood epilepsy or benign epilepsy

Discussion

This condition accounts for about 16% of childhood epilepsy. The family history of epilepsy in first degree relatives is positive in about 30%. Seizures may be simple partial, especially in daytime, or generalised tonic-clonic, especially in sleep.

Treatment depends of the number of seizures as with or without treatment spontaneous remission typically occurs before the age of 15 years and outlook for future scholastic achievement is good.

EEG

Background is normal
Interictal shows unilateral and/or bilateral blunt high amplitude centrotemporal spikes.

Question 8

a) Partially treated bacterial meningitis

Typical CSF findings after first year of life:

Diagnosis	*Cells/mm³*	*Protein g/l*	*Glucose mmol/l*
Normal	0–5, lymphocytes	0.2–0.4	2.8-4.8
Bacterial	200–2,000 (PMN)	Increased	Very low
Viral	100–1,000 (lymphocytes)	N/↑ 0.45-0.85	N (↓ in mumps)
TB	100–1,000 (lymphocytes)	↑ 0.6-5.0	↓ 0.5-2.0

Question 9

a)   Increase the I:E ratio
     Increase the Peak Airway Pressure

These two manoeuvres increase the mean airway pressure.

Question 10

a)   Distal renal tubular acidosis (type I)
b)   Hereditary
     Idiopathic
     Ehlers Danlos
     Amphotericin
     Hypercalcaemia
     Hypokalaemia
c)   Shohl's solution – potassium and sodium citrate
     Nephrolithotomy

This is hyperchloraemic (normal anion gap) acidosis with hypokalaemia. Renal tubular acidosis is caused by abnormalities in renal regulation of bicarbonate. Patients with this type of RTA may present with unexplained acidosis, failure to thrive, hypokalaemia, or one of the complications such as nephrolithiasis, nephrocalcinosis, rickets or polyuria. The urine pH does not fall below 6. Hypokalaemia is common and may be severe. Hypercalciuria is common and urinary citrate excretion is low.

Administration of alkali in the form of sodium bicarbonate or sodium citrate, the latter usually given as Shohl's solution which contains 1 mmol of citrate per ml of solution. A proportion of the alkali can be given as potassium bicarbonate or citrate.

EXAM 3 : CASE HISTORIES

Case History 1

a) Acute lymphoblastic leukaemia
b) Bone marrow biopsy
   Peripheral blood film

Key Points
- A multisystem disease with several features in the history:
  - a) Bleeding disorder - unexplained bruise
  - b) Fever and sore throat
  - c) Painless lymphadenopathy
  - d) Spinal cord lesion in the lumbar region
  - e) Possible meningitis - stiff neck and back
- Acute lymphoblastic leukaemia with meningeal infiltration is the most likely explanation.

Discussion

Acute leukaemia is the commonest malignant condition of childhood, the leukaemias together accounting for 30% of childhood cancers.
About 70% are acute lymphoblastic (ALL), 20% acute myeloblastic (AML) or variants.

Prognosis
ALL generally better than AML
Common and T cell better than B cell
High WBC > 60,000 carries poor prognosis
Age at presentation < 1 year or > 14 years poor prognosis
Presence of CNS involvement at diagnosis is an unfavourable feature
Prognosis is better if remission achieved within 14 days of induction

Overall survival 75%.

Case History 2

a) Blocked endotracheal tube
Displaced endotracheal tube
Pneumothorax requiring drainage
Ventilator failure

Key Points
- This question aims to establish whether the candidate has practical experience of working in a neonatal unit.
- The question is quite specific in describing a rapidly correctable situation and so intraventricular haemorrhage and sepsis would be incorrect answers.
- As neonatology achieves a higher profile in paediatrics, so the number of questions devoted to neonatology will increase.

Case History 3

a)   Visit to a forest or foreign land
b)   Serum specific IgM to *Borrelia burgdorferi*
c)   Penicillin; tetracycline is contraindicated because of the effect on growing teeth

Erythema chronicum migrans, most common manifestation of Lyme disease, begins usually 4 to 20 days after the bite of an *ixodid* tick. An erythematous macule forms gradually enlarging to form a plaque-like, erythematous annular lesion of median diameter 16 cm. The usual sites include the thigh, buttocks and axillae. Half the patients have multiple secondary annular lesions. The average duration of the untreated lesion is 3 weeks. The rash may be confused with streptococcal cellulitis, erythema multiforme (when multiple) or erythema marginatum. Often, ECM is associated with systematic symptoms such as malaise, fatigue, headache, stiff neck and arthralgia. Fever is usually low grade but may be as high as 40°C. Regional lymphadenopathy, anicteric hepatitis, conjunctivitis or pharyngitis may also occur. These symptoms usually resolve over several days but may be intermittent over several weeks.

Neurological involvement usually occurs within four weeks of the tick bite. Meningitis, cranial nerve palsies and peripheral neuropathy are most common, whilst meningoencephalitis, Guillain-Barré syndrome, pseudo-tumour cerebri and myelitis may also occur. Cardiac abnormalities occur more commonly in young adult males. Arthritis has been described in the USA but rarely in the UK.

The diagnosis is made on clinical and epidemiological grounds and confirmed by specific serology. The organism may be isolated from blood or cerebrospinal fluid.

Reference
Shapiro ED, *Tick-borne diseases*, Advances in Pediatric Infectious Diseases, 13:187-218, 1997.

Case History 4

a) Meconium ileus equivalent
   Intussusception
   Appendix abscess
b) Gastrografin enema

Discussion

Meconium ileus can produce intestinal obstruction in cystic fibrosis at any time from neonatal (or uterine) to adult life. In the initial stages either 50 ml oral gastrografin or acetylcysteine 5 ml tds may relieve the obstruction. A gastrografin enema, provided the patient is stable with no signs of perforation or dehydration, can be both diagnostic and therapeutic.

Where presumptive cases of meconium ileus equivalent fail to respond to the above measures, intussusception must be considered and surgery may be necessary.

Case History 5

a) Guillain-Barré syndrome/Ascending polyneuritis
b) Lumbar puncture
c) Serial vital captivity

Key Points
- The past history of meningitis is irrelevant
- Expressionless face is a clue to the facial weakness
- Be precise in answering the question

Discussion

A 3 day history of limb weakness, facial weakness and double vision with absent peripheral reflexes. The imminent danger is of respiratory muscle involvement with consequent respiratory failure.

Lumbar puncture may show cyto-albumin dissociation. Nerve conduction studies are of assistance in making the diagnosis at an early stage. The differential diagnosis would be myasthenia gravis.

EXAM 3 : DATA INTERPRETATIONS

Question 1

a)   Pyloric stenosis causing hypochloraemic alkalosis

Question 2

a)   Less than 1%
b)   1 in 50,000

Four fifths of achondroplastics are new genetic mutations, born to unaffected parents. Although neither parent is affected, the risk of having another affected child is above that of the general population as one of the parents may exhibit gonadal mosaicism.

Question 3

a)   Nesidioblastosis

Note the markedly elevated and inappropriate insulin level and absence of ketones. Hypoglycaemia may usefully be considered in terms of the presence of ketonuria. The former implies lack of substrate and the latter a hyperinsulinaemia state.

Nesidioblastosis is the most common hyperinsulinaemia state and presents usually in the first weeks or months of life. There is disordered islet cell organisation and a relative somatostatin deficiency allowing an inappropriate rise in insulin levels (normal $\leq$ 10 mU/1 when blood glucose <2.5 mmol/l).

Hypoglycaemia in hyperinsulinism may require intravenous dextrose infusion at rates up to 20 mg/kg/min. There is no response to glucagon. Diazoxide inhibits insulin secretion and subtotal pancreatectomy may be required if this fails.

Question 4

a)   Obstructive airways disease
     Increased residual volume
     Reversibility
b)   Whole body plethysmography
     Helium dilution

Discussion

Obstructive lung disease is often defined as reversible if, following administration of a bronchodilator, there is a 15% improvement in FEV_1. Airways disease accelerates the increase in residual volume. Any airways narrowing or loss of recoil, allowing dynamic compression, facilitates air trapping within the lungs and hence an increased residual volume is a characteristic feature of obstructive airways disease.

The total lung capacity depends on the balance of the ability of the respiratory muscles to expand the chest and the tendency of the lungs and chest wall to recoil inward towards their resting position. The increase in lung disease is due primarily to the loss of elastic recoil, often related to localised damage with lung cysts or bullae.

Question 5

a) Karyotype
    Thyroid function tests
b) Primary hypothyroidism
c) Thyroxine replacement therapy, a marked personality change may
    occur in the child

Delayed bone age and declining height velocity are firm reasons to investigate this girl's short stature. Turner's syndrome and hypothyroidism should be considered in any teenage girl who presents in this way, even if the clinical features are not obvious.

In a standard insulin tolerance test there should be an appropriate hypoglycaemia, GH should rise to exceed 12.5, cortisol should double its base level. FSH/LH should rise in parallel to GnRH challenge. In this example, the GH response is borderline low but the most striking abnormality is the very high baseline TSH which is unresponsive to TRH implying that this is primary organ associated hypothyroidism

Thyroxine replacement therapy should be commenced with great care because of its effects on the cardiovascular system. Progress should be monitored symptomatically and by the TSH level. Parents should be warned that a previously inactive docile child will become more energetic and her school performance may also suffer until stabilisation is attained.

Question 6

a)   Complete atrio-ventricular conduction block (heart block)

Question 7

a)   Leukaemia
     Systematic lupus erythematosus

Pancytopenia with haematuria may be due to marrow replacement or suppression. Nephritis may also be present in SLE. Aplastic anaemia is another possible answer.

Question 8

a)   Kawasaki disease
b)   Echocardiogram
c)   Intravenous gammaglobulin 400mg/kg/d and oral aspirin, high dose until fever settles then low dose thereafter.

Criteria for diagnosis:

1)   Persistent high fever for at least five days
2)   Bilateral conjuctival injection
3)   Pleomorphic rash
4)   Swelling and induration of hands and feet
5)   Desquamation of fingers and toes
6)   Cervical lymphadenopathy

Strict case definition requires the presence of at least five of the six criteria, or four plus coronary artery aneurysms. With the help of echocardiography however, Kawasaki disease is being diagnosed with increasing frequency in patients with 3 or fewer of the major signs.

Question 9

a)   4–4 ½ years
b)   Formal testing of hearing

Discussion

Shapes
Children can imitate before they can copy a shape, so read the question carefully. From 3 years children are generally asked to copy shapes.

	50th centile	90th centile
Vertical line	2 ½ years	3 years
Circle	2 years 9 months	3 ½ years
Cross	4 years	4 years 8 months
Square	4 years 7 months	5 years 3 months
Triangle	5 years	5 ½ years

Hearing and language
At 4 years most children can count to ten without a mistake. By 3 years 5 months 90% of children can give their first and family name. Failure in these aspects may represent developmental delay or psychosocial deprivation. The most important initial step is to test this child's hearing formally. A speech discrimination test would be useful as an initial screen, although free field audiometry would be more precise.

Question 10

a) Reticulocyte count
   Bone marrow examination
   Blood film
b) Diamond-Blackfan syndrome/Pure red cell aplasia

The baby's anaemia is not due to Rhesus or ABO incompatibility. The white count and platelets are normal. Diamond-Blackfan syndrome usually presents with profound anaemia by 2 to 6 months. The most important diagnostic feature is the absence of red cell precursors in blood and bone marrow. Erythropoietin levels are high.

Treatment is supportive with transfusions and steroids. A few cases remit spontaneously, otherwise death occurs in the second decade without bone marrow transplantation.

EXAM 4 : CASE HISTORIES

Case History 1

a)   Pulmonary hypertension
b)   Atrial fibrillation
c)   Pulmonary embolism

A loud second (presumed pulmonary) heart sound accompanied by diastolic murmur signifies pulmonary hypertension with functional valvular incompetence. This is a serious complication of a systematic-pulmonary shunt. Pulmonary embolism is a well known consequence of atrial fibrillation. Endocarditis should be borne in mind in questions of this nature. Patch detachment is an early complication.

Case History 2

a)   Septic screen including lumbar puncture
     Blood glucose
     Serum calcium and electrolytes
b)   Drug withdrawal

Key Points
- Several classical features of withdrawal – jitteriness, temperature instability, sweatiness, tachycardia. Feeding disturbance such as increased demand and disordered suck occurs.
- In this case the feeding history makes severe sepsis unlikely
- Note also the unbooked pregnancy and the absence of antenatal information

Discussion

Drug withdrawal is increasingly commonly seen. Symptoms also include diarrhoea, apnoea, rhinorrhea, and convulsions and may start at any time in the first two weeks. Methadone, a heroine substitute, causes a period of withdrawal lasting up to three months. Withdrawal can be suppressed with chlorpromazine or diazepam (small doses of morphine in U.S.A.) reducing over several weeks. Drug abuse in the mother should prompt investigation of the social situation and exclusion of HIV and Hepatitis B.

Case History 3

a)   ASOT 1,200 I.U.
b)   Sydenham's chorea
c)   Penicillin
d)   Usually normal

Key Points
- The abnormal movements described are choreiform. The possible differential is stereotypy which consists of the same movement repeated, usually sparing the face.
- Absence of family history or drug ingestion (neuroleptics, phenytoin)
- The story of a fright is irrelevant and the 'old council house' is a false clue for lead poisoning

Discussion

The onset of Sydenham's chorea is usually insidious, more common in girls with fidgetiness, frowning, head and eye rolling, slurred speech, jerky respiration and exaggerated uncoordinated movements. All abnormal movements are made worse by excitement and cease in sleep. Mental state may be labile. Cardiac disease may be present but usually there is no fever or signs of rheumatic fever.

Investigations aim to prove the presence of streptococcal infection and search for other organ damage.

Treatment traditionally includes bed rest, a course of penicillin and prophylaxis until adult life, psychological and physiotherapy support, and follow up, if appropriate, for cardiac disease.

Reference
Heye N, Jergas M, Hotzinger H et al, *Sydenham's chorea: Clinical, EEG, MRI and SPECT findings in the early stage of the disease*, Journal of Neurology, 240(2):121-3, 1993 Feb.

Case History 4

a) Thyroid function tests
b) Untreated at 10 weeks
   Both parents of low intelligence

Congenital hypothyroidism has an incidence of 1 in 3,000, three times as common in girls as in boys. It has recently been demonstrated that thyroid hormones can cross the placenta, hence infants are not frankly 'cretinous' at birth. It is possible that one or both parents are also affected. Hirschsprung's is associated. Feeding difficulties and nasal obstruction are typical. The temperature is subnormal and anaemia refractory to haematinics occurs.

Below are the clinical features described in congenital hypothyroidism*. Since the early signs are generally non-specific and the development of other features is slow, thyroid function tests should be performed in case of doubt.

Features which may be present at birth
Postmature, large size
Wide posterior fontanelle
Umbilical hernia
Goitre

Early signs, less than 4 weeks
Placid, 'good', sleeps a lot
Poor feeder
Constipation, abdominal distension
Mottled, cold
Oedema
Prolonged jaundice

Late signs
Cretinous appearance
Big tongue
Hoarse cry
Dry skin and hair
Slow responses
Retarded growth and development

(*Adapted from Robertson NRC. A Textbook of Neonatology. Churchill Livingstone)

The age at treatment and the genetic potential endowed by the parents limit the mental development. Patients in whom treatment is started before 6 weeks of age have an average IQ of 100. If treatment is started between 6 weeks and 3 months IQ drops to 95; between 3 and 6 months to 75; after 6 months, 55 or less.

Several other neurological deficits have been described including deafness, ataxia, attention deficit order, abnormal muscle tone and speech defects.

This question is a bit old fashioned as most children would be expected to have been detected at neonatal screening.

Case History 5

a) Coeliac disease
b) Jejunal biopsy for histological diagnosis

Key Points
- It is important not to be distracted by issues such as congenital heart disease or drug therapies
- Congenital heart disease is responsible for poor growth in some circumstances, dioxin overdose may cause nausea and vomiting but the question asks for the most likely cause.
- Contained in this question is a classical description of a child presenting with coeliac disease

Discussion

Coeliac disease is a gluten induced enteropathy requiring characteristic histological findings to confirm the diagnosis. Increasing use is being made of specific antibody tests, IgG and IgA antigliadin and antiendomyseal antibodies. In the future, use of these antibody tests and a good response to a gluten free diet may obviate the need for further challenge biopsy. Transient gluten intolerance is more common under one year of age and a gluten challenge should be conducted after one year on a gluten free diet. Other causes of a similar biopsy appearance of total villous atrophy include giardiasis, post-enteritis enteropathy and tropical sprue.

EXAM 4 : DATA INTERPRETATIONS

Question 1

a) Intestinal lymphangiectasia
b) Jejunal biopsy
   Chromium labelled albumin studies

Discussion

There are a number of mechanisms in protein losing enteropathies.

a)	Exudation from ulcerative or inflammatory lesion	e.g. Crohn's; U.C. Intestinal T.B.
b)	Defective lymphatic drainage	e.g. Intestinal lymphagangiectasia; neoplasia affecting mesenteric lymphatics
c)	Unknown	e.g. Coeliac disease; Henoch-Schönlein purpura

The diagnosis is made by first excluding cirrhosis and nephrotic syndrome. Confirmation is by demonstrating excess faecal loss of ^{51}Cr labelled albumin. In this particular case the history and investigations suggest a specific diagnosis. Intestinal lymphagiectasia presents in childhood, oedema usually preceding diarrhoea. The characteristic lesion seen on biopsy is dilation of the small bowel lymphatics. There is always a marked hypoalbuminaemia and all immunoglobulins are also reduced. The peripheral white count is always abnormal with severe reduction of lymphocytes. Treatment is generally supportive with medium chain triglycerides which are more easily absorbed than normal dietary fat.

Question 2

a) X linked recessive
b) Nil
c) 1 in 4

Question 3

a) Encephalitis
b) Herpes simplex virus

Question 4

a) Inorganic lead encephalopathy
b) Free red cell protoporphyrin
    Urine coproporphyrin
    Blood (lead)

There are signs of encephalopathy, anaemia, proteinuria and glycosuria. Lead causes proximal renal tubular damage and by interfering with iron utilisation and haemoglobin synthesis causes hypochromic, microcytic anaemia.

Question 5

a) Profound bilateral sensori-neural hearing loss
b) Pneumococcal meningitis

Following the new HiB vaccination programme *H. influenzae* is now rarely seen. Pneumococcal meningitis is the most likely to cause such severe deafness.

Note also that:

- Only unmasks bone conduction is obtainable in severe binaural disease
- The air bone gap at 250 and 500 Hz is false at these frequencies at levels around 50 dBHL bone conduction thresholds are felt through vibration, 'vibration thresholds'
- Bone conduction thresholds are only measurable 'down' to 60 dBHL and the presence of a false air-bone gap therefore appears in severe or profound losses

Question 6

a) Supraventricular tachycardia

b) IV adenosine or DC cardioversion

Childhood SVT is associated with a small risk of death. Infants especially tolerate tachycardia less well than adults as they are more dependent on heart rate for cardiac output and have fewer reserves.

Ventricular tachycardia should be excluded. If the child is sick, the child should have DC cardioversion with full resuscitative facilities at hand. However, if the child is tolerating the tachycardia and it is judged to be a junctional tachycardia, a vagal manoeuvre may be successful. This may compromise immersion of the face in cold water, blowing on the face or unilateral cartoid sinus massage.

If vagal manoeuvres fail, intravenous adenosine is the drug of choice. It acts by slowing AV nodal conduction, thus disrupting re-entry circuits. It is effective within 10–15 seconds of administration and has a half life of the same order. Unlike verapamil it is not negatively inotropic in this form. It has a high safety profile, its main drawback being the fact that 30% of tachycardias will reinitiate.

If adenosine fails, the diagnosis should be reconsidered and if the child is still well, a second line drug such as intravenous flecainide tried. Otherwise DC cardioversion, initially 1J/kg, with a short acting anaesthetic, is an option.

Question 7

a) Infectious mononucleosis
b) Serology for specific Epstein-Barr IgM antibody

Discussion

Clinical presentation of infectious mononucleosis is variable:

General features:	Fever, lymphadenopathy, pharyngitis, splenomegaly (50%), mild hepatomegaly, jaundice
Cardiac:	Myocarditis, arrhythmias
Neurological:	Aseptic meningitis, cranial nerve palsies, transverse myelitis
Haematological:	Atypical monocytes 5–50% total white cell count, actually transformed T cells
	Auto-immune haemolytic anaemia with cold agglutinins
	Thrombocytopenia

Investigations:

The heterophile antibody test (Paul Bunnell) is occasionally negative in early stages of infectious mononucleosis and may also give false-positive results. Specific IgM antibody to EBV indicates a very recent or current infection.

Question 8

a) Commence anticonvulsants
b) Serum calcium, CT brain scan
Blood culture
Urine culture
c) Idiopathic epilepsy
Febrile convulsions
Subarachnoid haemorrhage in view of the blood stained CSF

This infant has had 3 convulsions in the space of a few hours. This may be the presentation of idiopathic epilepsy or simple febrile convulsions, although it should be noted that she is quite young for the latter. Alternatively, we are not told whether the lumbar puncture was traumatic or not, raising the possibility of an intracranial haemorrhage.

Question 9

a) Coarctation of the aorta
Ventricular septal defect
Patent ductus arteriosus

Discussion

Working through each chamber sequentially as previously outlined, there is a significant step-up in saturation at right ventricular level, indicating a left to right shunt. The step down at aortic level confirms a right to left shunt via a patent ductus arteriosus.

The history describes a preductal (infantile) coarctation, in which persistence of the ductus arteriosus is a common feature. The descending aorta receives most of its blood supply from the main pulmonary artery via the ductus arteriosus, while the left ventricle continues to supply the first two or three aortic branches. The pulmonary hypertension initially accompanies a high pulmonary blood flow, but may later reflect increasing pulmonary resistance.

In preductal coarctation, congestive cardiac failure is often precipitated in the earliest days or weeks of life. If possible, the preductal segment is excised and either end-to-end anastomosis or subclavian patch repair performed, followed by surgical closure of the ductus arteriosus.

Question 10

a)   Anaemia of prematurity

Discussion

The cause of this anaemia is multifactorial. Following the rise in pO_2 after delivery, erythropoietin levels fall and become undetectable in the plasma for 1 to 2 months. In both full term and premature infants the haemoglobin level falls, and in premature infants may fall to 7–8g/dl during the second month. The red cell lifespan in premature infants is of the order of two weeks. This fall is mirrored by a reticulocyte count of about 4% at birth which falls to 1–2% during the first month.

Folic acid deficiency and vitamin E deficiency may both play a part in anaemia of prematurity but iron deficiency is not important in the early stage.

In this case the reticulocyte response is satisfactory and the haemoglobin usually begins to rise slowly and transfusion is not required.

EXAM 5 : CASE HISTORIES

Case History 1

a)   Biliary colic
b)   Abdominal ultrasound

Key Points
- Intermittent pain commencing after mealtimes suggests biliary colic
- He is comfortable on examination and the pain is settling. The steady haemoglobin value excludes two important differentials in sickle cell disease:

Hepatic sequestration
occurs in all age groups
abdominal distension with severe hypochondrial pain
rapidly enlarging tense liver

Girdle syndrome
silent distended abdomen
hepatic enlargement common
often bilateral basal lung consolidation

Discussion

30% of children and 70% of adults with sickle cell disease have gallstones. These are often asymptomatic but can cause
acute cholecystitis
chronic cholangitis
biliary colic
obstruction at the common bile duct
related acute pancreatis

As many as 50% of stones may be radiopaque so may be visible on plain abdominal X-ray. Ultrasound of gall bladder or oral cholecystogram are most likely to confirm the diagnosis.
Acute cholecystitis is managed with analgesia, hydration and antibiotics. If recurrent problems occur then elective open or laparoscopic cholecystectomy may be necessary, with careful pre-operative preparation often with exchange transfusion.

Case History 2

a)   Full blood count including packed cell volume
     Clotting studies
b)   Fresh frozen plasma

Key Points
- There is no record that this baby received Vitamin K after birth and this was probably missed in the ambulance and forgotten after admission
- The sticky stools suggest gastrointestinal haemorrhage
- Testing the stool for blood is a reasonable answer, but since only two tests are allowed, blood count and clotting are more important

Discussion

Haemorrhagic disease of the newborn has a significant mortality. Vitamin K even given intravenously does not act immediately and fresh frozen plasma should be given to replace deficient clotting factors.

Following the recent controversy over the link between vitamin K and childhood cancer, it is likely that more cases like this will occur. BPA recommendations suggest 3 doses of vitamin K orally are as effective as IM treatment, but compliance is then more likely to be a problem.

Case History 3

a) CT brain scan or cerebral angiography
b) Sagittal sinus thrombosis
   Encephalitis or meningitis with raised intracranial pressure

Key Points
- Clinical history of severe dehydration, but a full anterior fontanelle suggests raised intracranial pressure. Normal fundi do not exclude this.
- Note elevated CSF protein value (see normal values).
- The question is specific in asking for investigations to confirm a diagnosis, not immediate investigation, so electrolytes would not be an appropriate answer.

Discussion

Thrombosis of the cerebral veins occurs principally as a complication of severe dehydration, or as an extension of local infection. Sagittal sinus thrombosis occurs mainly in infants who are severely dehydrated often as a consequence of diarrhoea, although one hopes with increasing understanding of oral rehydration therapy it will become less common. The venous obstruction leads to cerebral swelling with signs of raised intracranial pressure including stupor, coma and bulging anterior fontanelle. Seizures and quadriparesis may occur, often with involvement of the extremities first.

Clinically, the condition may mimic encephalitis and metabolic encephalopathy. Practically, if there is ever a suspicion of raised intracranial pressure a lumbar puncture should not be performed; normal fundi do not exclude intracranial pressure.

A CT scan may show the area of thrombosis, often with widespread haemorrhagic infarction of the brain. Cerebral angiography is of value in localising the site of obstruction. CSF examination is of little help, but pressure is normally elevated, the fluid may be bloody and show white cells and an elevated protein content.

Apart from supportive management, streptokinase infusion may have a role to play although research with this drug has mainly been in adults.

Case History 4

a)   Sweat test
     Nasal brushings for ciliary function
     Immunoglobulins
b)   Primary ciliary dyskinesia

Key Points
   - All the information in this question is relevant, do not miss points like 'thriving'
   - It is important not to dismiss information such as the presence of serous otitis media as a 'red herring', rather consider it in the context of the differential diagnosis

Discussion

A number of conditions with abnormalities of ciliary function are now recognised.

Kartagener's classically implies situs inversus, sinusitis and bronchiectasis and is autosomal recessive with incomplete penetrance. Only half of primary ciliary dyskinesia cases have situs inversus.

As the condition is present from birth, these patients have a history of respiratory distress at birth. Later chronic upper and lower respiratory tract disease is almost universal. There is a strong correlation with secretory otitis media and conductive hearing loss.

Diagnosis requires nasal brushings and immediate motility studies by photometric means. Electron microscopy shows a wide variety of structural defects including defective dynein arms or missing spokes.

As the problem is a structural one it is irreversible and so treatment is aimed at delaying the onset and progression of bronchiectasis with antibiotics and physiotherapy. Hearing should be tested and ENT intervention sought if appropriate. Many males are infertile and appropriate sperm mobility tests and counselling should be carried out.

Reference
Corbeel L et al, *Ultrastructural abnormalities of bronchial cilia in children with recurrent airway infections and bronchiectasis,* Archives of Disease in Childhood. 56(12):929-33, 1981 Dec.

Case History 5

a)   Subdural haematoma
b)   Skeletal survey
       CT brain scan
       Clotting studies
c)   Liase with Child Protection Team

Discussion

CT scan adds information about the timing of the haemorrhage. As the haematoma resolves, the appearance of blood changes from a hyperdense to an ultimately hypodense appearance.

A repeated shaking injury can lead to subdural haematoma in the absence of external signs of injury to the head. Cerebral bridging veins are torn at their fixed attachments to sagittal sutures.

The site, age and nature of the haemorrhage all assist in the diagnosis. All children suspected of having intracranial haemorrhage should have a CT scan.

In cases of child abuse, the clinical and pathological features should be viewed in the family context. In determining a course of action, the importance of parental responsibility and the child's own wishes are emphasised in the Children Act.

Reference
Hobbs CJ, *Skull fracture and the diagnosis of abuse,* Archives of Disease in Childhood. 59(3):246-52, 1984 Mar.

EXAM 5 : DATA INTERPRETATIONS

Question 1

a) Hypokalaemic alkalosis
b) Renin or aldosterone
c) Bartter's syndrome

Question 2

a) Autosomal recessive or X-linked recessive
b) Autosomal recessive
c) Approximately 98%

Discussion

The incidence of congenital hearing loss (greater than 50 dB) in Western Europe is approximately 1:1,000 live births. In at least 50% of cases the cause is generic and may be syndromic, autosomal recessive or X-linked recessive. The most common inheritance pattern is autosomal recessive but at least 15 gene loci may be involved in the causation of non-syndromic autosomal recessive hearing loss. The chance of Family A and Family B sharing the same gene defect is small but in absence of more information an empirical recurrence rate of 12% may be quoted.

Question 3

a) Short PR interval
   Delta wave
b) Symptomatic tachycardia

The most common arrythmias are a regular atrio-ventricular re-entrant tachycardia and atrial fibrillation, both which cause symptoms and carry the risk of sudden death.

Question 4

a)   Conn's syndrome
     Cushing's syndrome
     Renal artery stenosis
     Congenital adrenal hyperplasia
     Diuretic abuse

Any of these would fit the electrolyte pattern.

Question 5

a)   Williams' syndrome
b)   Supravalvular aortic stenosis

Discussion

It is important to be precise with this answer and aortic stenosis alone would not score full marks. Williams' syndrome is of unknown aetiology and is associated with hypercalcaemia in infancy.

Cardiac	Supravalvular aortic stenosis
	Peripheral pulmonary artery stenosis
	Pulmonary valve stenosis
Facial	Prominent 'fish' lips
	Blue eyes with stellate pattern in iris
	Short palpebral fissures
Neuro	Developmental delay
	Mild microcephaly

These children tend to be lively and cope well with verbal and social skills but have delayed motor and perceptual abilities. Average IQ 50.

Question 6

a)   7 years
b)   Yes

Discussion

Again the question states copy not imitate. These shapes are from the modified Binet and Bender-Gestalt test, and most are used in the Griffith's mental development scales.

By 7 years most children can write their own name.

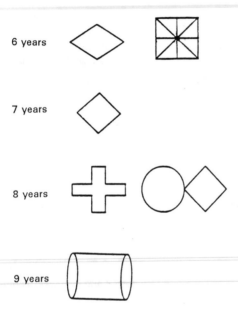

6 years

7 years

8 years

9 years

Question 7

a)   Critical pulmonary stenosis
b)   Prostaglandin E2
c)   Balloon dilation of pulmonary artery

Question 8

a) ABO incompatibility
b) Maternal anti-A haemolysin

Note that the reticulocyte count is normal for a neonate and that spherocytes are seen in many cases of haemolysis. The positive indirect Coomb's test implies the presence of antibodies.

Question 9

a) Whooping cough

Discussion

Causative organism *Bordetella pertussis*. May be cultured in early cases from a nasopharyngeal swab in Border-Gengou medium, but is very difficult to isolate once the cough is established.

Diagnosis is largely clinical but a striking absolute lymphocytosis supports the diagnosis.

Serology for complement fixating antibodies. These are nearly always present by the third week.

Complications include bronchopneumonia, bronchiectasis, convulsions and subconjunctival haemorrhages.

Question 10

a) Congenital cyanotic heart disease with right to left shunt

If a normal infant is given more than 80% FiO_2 for more than 10 minutes, the arterial pO_2 should exceed 20 kPa. If pO_2 is below this level, cyanotic heart disease may be present. This is unlikely above 20 kPa and excluded above 27 kPa.

EXAM 6 : CASE HISTORIES

Case History 1

a) Juvenile myoclonic epilepsy
b) Sleep EEG (EEG alone would score, but fewer marks)
c) Prescribe sodium valproate as anti-epileptic drug of choice

Key Points

- Juvenile myoclonic epilepsy (JME) is a primary generalised epilepsy usually presenting between 8 and 18 years of age.
- A history of early morning myoclonus is crucial. This normally precedes any generalised tonic clonic seizure, and the symptom is usually described by patients as clumsiness and dropping things.
- Seizures are especially likely to be provoked by consumption of alcohol or sleep deprivation.
- The EEG is characteristic with multiple spikes and slow waves. Brain imaging is normal but is not necessary for the diagnosis.
- Most patients are well controlled on sodium valproate monotherapy but Lamotrigine is also effective both as monotherapy and as adjunctive therapy.

References

Aicardi J, *Diseases of the Nervous System in Childhood,* Clinics in Developmental Medicine No 115/118 1992, MacKeith Press, Oxford.

Case History 2

a) Group B Streptococcal septicaemia
b) Meconium aspiration syndrome
c) Prolonged rupture of membranes
   Maternal pyrexia
   Maternal Group B Streptococcal colonisation
d) Antibiotics
   Penicillin & gentamicin (best answer)
   Fresh frozen plasma (fewer marks)
   Blood transfusion with packed cells (fewer marks)
   Intra-venous immunoglobulin (fewer marks)

Key Points
- Prolonged rupture of membranes (Note 'PROM' and all abbreviations should be avoided, as they may not score marks)
- Maternal pyrexia
- Thrombocytopenia, anaemia, deranged clotting all suggests sepsis
- Meconium passage suggests fetal distress

Discussion

Group B Streptococcus is a major cause of neonatal morbidity and mortality. Maternal colonisation rates vary with different populations and regions. Infected newborns may present with overwhelming sepsis and shock from birth or present up to 6 weeks later with, for example, pneumonia or meningitis. Benzylpenicillin and Gentamicin are recognised first line antibiotics which should be considered in every neonate who presents with signs of possible sepsis. Adjunctive treatment such as intravenous immunoglobulin has been used in some centres but its effectiveness in robust clinical trials has not yet been proven.

Reference
Isaacs D, *Prevention of early onset Group B Streptococcal Infection: Screen, treat or observe.* Arch Dis Child Foetal and neonatal edition 1998 **79**; 81–82

Case History 3

a) Cows' milk protein intolerance
b) Colonoscopy and biopsy and small intestinal biopsy
c) IgE level and serum RAST for milk protein may be positive. Skin prick test to cows' milk

Key Points

- Symptoms in first 12 months of life
- Children can be sensitized even if breast-fed
- Enteropathy not invariably present, and is patchy with flat mucosa
- If colitis is the presenting feature, colonoscopy may show eosinophilic colitis

Discussion

Onset of cows' milk protein intolerance may be acute or chronic. Acute anaphylaxis occurs in some infants. The chronic onset group may manifest as chronic diarrhoea with failure to thrive and clinical features to suggest coeliac disease. It has been shown that infants can be sensitized to cows' milk through maternal breast milk when the mother is drinking cows' milk.

Raised IgE and positive RAST to cows' milk as well as a positive skin prick test (usually in the acute onset group) to cows' milk help confirm the diagnosis of cows' milk allergy. Biopsy of the proximal intestinal mucosa is often abnormal at the time of initial diagnosis. Cows' milk protein intolerance causes a patchy enteropathy. Cows' milk colitis is characterised by an eosinophilic colitis.

Protein hydrolysate feeds (e.g. Nutramigen) or amino acid formula (e.g Neocate) are preferred for cows' milk protein intolerance as such children can be sensitised to soya protein as well.

Reference
Walker-Smith, Hamilton, *Practical Paediatric Gastroenterology*, 2nd ed. p188-191, BC Decker.

Case History 4

a) Pauciarticular juvenile chronic arthritis
b) Antinuclear antibodies
c) Slit lamp examination of the eyes

Key Points
- Pauciarticular type 1 mainly affects girls under the age of 4
- Rheumatoid factor negative
- If ANA positive, high risk for iridocyclitis

Discussion

Juvenile chronic arthritis is defined as arthritis of more than 3 months duration. Girls are predominantly affected, and the disease generally begins before age 4. Patients with iridocyclitis frequently have positive tests for antinuclear antibodies. Children may note redness of the eyes, pain or photophobia, although it can develop asymptomatically. Therefore regular ophthalmological assessment is essential.

Reference
Woo P. et al, *Juvenile Chronic Arthritis,*
Lancet, 1998 Mar 28;351 (9107):969-73, Review.

Case History 5

a) Hereditary angioedema
b) C1 Esterase inhibitor levels
c) C1 inhibitor concentrate or fresh frozen plasma

Key Points
- Inability to synthesise normally functioning C1 inhibitor
- 85% have very low levels of inhibitor
- 15% have normal or raised non-functioning protein
- Both forms autosomal dominant inheritance

Discussion

Angioedema is a type of urticaria, which characterisically involves the deeper layers of skin or submucosa. Hereditary angioedema accounts for 2% of all cases of angioedema. Viral illness, trauma, menses and emotional stress can trigger an attack. Swelling of the intestinal wall can lead to intense abdominal cramping, sometimes with diarrhoea and vomiting. Concurrent subcutaneous oedema may be absent. Laryngeal oedema can be fatal. For acute life-threatening attacks, C1 Esterase concentrates or FFP are required, as steroids, adrenaline and antihistamines are not effective in this situation. Danazol increases serum levels of C1 Esterase inhibitor and may be used for short-term and long-term prophylaxis. However, long-term use may lead to androgenic problems in children.

Reference
Borum M L, *Hereditary Angioedema. Complex symptoms can make diagnosis difficult,* Postgrad Med 1998 Apr; 103(4):251.255-6.

EXAM 6 : DATA INTERPRETATIONS

Question 1

a) Oropharyngeal airway
    Administer facial oxygen
    Prone nursing
b) Pierre-Robin Syndrome

Key Points
* Pierre-Robin syndrome is micrognathia with glossoptosis and high arched or cleft palate
* Airway management by positioning can obviate need for intubation

Discussion

Although this baby has marked respiratory acidosis, the need for intubation and ventilation may be avoided by maintaining the airway. Babies with Pierre-Robin Syndrome can obstruct their airway with the tongue falling back, under the influence of gravity. Nursing in the prone position may alleviate the problem, by allowing the tongue to fall forward. If the clinical condition and blood gas do not show rapid improvement with these manoeuvres then nasal cPAP or intubation and ventilation will be necessary. Often the growth of the mandible will achieve a more normal profile by 4–6 years.

Question 2

a) Poor/non-compliance with therapy

Discussion

Far from being a 'trick question' this example demonstrates one of the most frequent causes of treatment failure. The psychological implications of diabetes in adolescence are not to be underestimated and non-compliance can become a major problem. The huge daily requirement for insulin is unusual in someone with no hypoglycaemic episodes, a high HBA1C and no injection site areas of lipoatrophy.

Question 3

a) Bone marrow biopsy for ring sideroblasts
b) Sideroblastic anaemia

Discussion

The differential diagnosis of a hypochromic anaemia includes the rarer but important group of congenital and acquired sideroblastic anaemias. In contrast to iron deficiency or thalassaemia, iron stores are raised, as is serum ferritin. Haemoglobin electrophoresis is of course normal. The hereditary form usually occurs in males and the acquired form can be primary or secondary to other malignant disease of the bone marrow and various drugs.

Question 4

a) 17 hydroxyprogesterone
b) Salt losing 21 hydroxylase deficiency form of congenital adrenal hyperplasia

Question 5

a) Partially compensated respiratory acidosis
b) Intubate and ventilate baby

Discussion

This is an acidosis because the pH is less than 7.3. Babies with chronic lung disease often run a relatively high pCO_2 (e.g. pCO_2 7 to 9). This is normally compensated by a high bicarbonate and base excess, so that the pH is in the normal range. The baby with chronic lung disease is particularly vulnerable to infections with RSV bronchiolitis, and in this case is deteriorating. The pCO_2 is raised even for chronic lung disease and the pH is below normal, making it an acidosis. It is partially compensated as the bicarbonate and base excess are raised, but insufficiently to normalise the pH.

Question 6

a) $2/3 \times 1/20 \times 1/4 = 1/120$
b) $1 \times 1/20 \times 1/2 = 1/40$

Key Points
- These are popular data questions.
- Don't forget that an unaffected sibling of a case with an autosomal recessive disease (such as cystic fibrosis) has a 2/3 probability of being a carrier for that disease.

Question 7

a) Subacute sclerosing panencephalitis
b) Raised measles antibody titres in the serum and CSF/Typical EEG changes with periodic and regular complexes

Key Points
- Cerebral changes many years after primary infection
- Insidious deterioration in higher cerebral function
- Elevated measles CSF antibody titre
- Periodic complexes on EEG

Discussion

This illness is rarely seen following the introduction of measles vaccine. School failure is often the first sign of subtle deterioration in higher cerebral function. Generalized myoclonic jerks at regular intervals are characteristic. The EEG typically shows repeated bursts of generalised high-voltage slow wave complexes, called periodic complexes. In this girl the electromyographic record shows associated myoclonus.

Question 8

a)   Central diabetes insipidus
b)   Cranial tuberculosis
c)   Intranasal DDAVP and anti-tuberculosis therapy

Key Points
- Dilute urine in face of high serum osmolality
- Paired serum and urine osmolality
- CT head
- Polyuria and polydipsia
- Water deprivation test aids diagnosis
- Classify type of diabetes insipidus
- Vasopressin levels are low in serum

Discussion

Central diabetes insipidus results from a lack of anti-diuretic hormone. Any lesion, which damages the neurohypophyseal unit, may cause DI. Encephalitis, tuberculosis, actinomycosis, and leukaemia are occasional causes. In a minority it is hereditary. In the newborn it may be due to intraventricular haemorrhage, group B streptococcal sepsis, DIC and asphyxia.

Compulsive water drinking or psychogenic polydipsia can be distinguished from diabetes insipidus as affected persons are able to produce concentrated urine when fluids are withheld.

In nephrogenic diabetes insipidus there is no response to DDAVP and vasopressin levels in serum and urine are normal.

DDAVP transiently increases factor VIII coagulant activity and is used before minor surgery in patients with von Willebrand's disease or mild haemophilia A.

Question 9

a) Juvenile dermatomyositis – heliotrope rash, proximal muscle weakness
b) EMG (electromyogram)
   Muscle biopsy
c) Prednisolone 1–2 mg/kg/day

Key Points
- Inflammation of smooth muscle and typical cutaneous lesions
- Occlusive vasculitis
- Raised transaminases, CK

Discussion

This is a multisystem disease characterised by inflammation of striated muscle, and typical cutaneous lesions. In muscle there is patchy degeneration, atrophy and regeneration. The most prominent lesion is an occlusive vasculitis. Myositis is predominant in proximal muscles.

The upper eyelids have a pathognomonic violaceous discoloration (heliotrope rash). Calcium may be deposited in affected subcutaneous tissues.

Rheumatoid factor and ANA are usually low or negative. The EMG of affected muscles is abnormal.

Severe involvement of the palato-respiratory muscles may affect breathing and in these children intubation and ventilation may be necessary.

Physiotherapy to avoid contractures, as well as steroid therapy, are the recommended treatments.

Question 10

a) Crohn's disease
b) Colonoscopy and biopsy
c) Enteral nutrition/steroids

Key Points
- Growth failure without GIT symptoms is a feature of childhood Crohn's disease
- Thrombocytosis is a sign of chronic inflammation
- Ferritin (iron stores) often depleted in Crohn's disease

CRP is a better marker of inflammation in Crohn's than ESR.

EXAM 7 : CASE HISTORIES

Case History 1

a) Marfan's Syndrome
b) Echocardiogram (best answer)
    Ophthalmological assessment (fewer marks)
c) Mitral valve prolapse with mitral regurgitation

Key Points

- This question is clearly describing phenotypic features of a recognised syndrome. You must be clear on diagnostic criteria for this and other syndromes including Prader-Willi, Angelman's, Fragile X, Williams' and of course Down's syndrome.
- Be careful to ensure that the cardiac lesion you describe will account for the physical signs described. Aortic root dilatation is common in Marfan's as is aortic incompetence, but this would not account for a pansystolic murmur.

Discussion

The most frequent musculoskeletal features at presentation are a combination of tall stature, limb disproportion, pectus deformity, classical facial features, high arched palate and arachnodactyly. During the pubertal growth spurt many children develop red striae distensae (stretch marks) and a scoliosis. Annual echocardiography is essential to defect early aortic root dilatation and monitor aortic root diameter. Ophthalmological assessment is also important to detect lens dislocation.

Reference
Lipscomb KJ, Clayton-Smith, Harris R. *Evolving phenotype of Marfan's syndrome.* Archives of Disease in Childhood 1997;**76**:41-46

Case History 2

a)   Nephritis secondary to systemic lupus erythematosus (nephritis alone would not score well)

b)   Renal biopsy and histology (this would be counted as one investigation)

c)   Oral prednisolone or IV high dose methylprednisolone
Cyclophosphamide or azathioprine

Key Points

- SLE and other connective tissue disorders have a variety of potential clinical presentations and so make good grey case questions! Absence of 'classical' butterfly rash in this case does not rule out the diagnosis.
- Renal biopsy is still the only way to confirm the diagnosis of lupus nephritis and histology will guide drug treatment.
- When asked for treatment of choice, always list the most commonly used treatments first. Then go on to list any other treatments. Although often only the first two or three treatments you list will receive marks, you will not have marks deducted for writing more.

Reference

White P.H. *Paediatric systemic lupus erythematosus and neonatal lupus.* Rheumatic Diseases Clinics of North America. 20(1):119-27, 1994.

Case History 3

a) Abdominal X-ray
b) Hirschsprung's disease – suction biopsy of the rectum
c) Hirschsprung's enterocolitis

Discussion

In Hirschsprung's disease, AXR may show dilated loops of large and small bowel with no air in the rectum, and signs of intestinal obstruction. It is important to realise that breast-fed babies can have a wide variation in their bowel frequency – from stool with virtually every feed, to once per week. Cows' milk is known to be associated with constipation, but this baby did not respond to cows' milk exclusion.

To make the diagnosis of Hirschsprung's, a rectal biopsy needs to be performed and the tissue stained for acetylcholine for the presence of ganglion cells. These are absent in Hirschsprung's. Although it is important to ask about meconium passage in the first 24 hours, this is not always delayed in Hirschsprung's. Hirschsprung's enterocolitis may present with an acute abdomen, shock and rectal bleeding. This is a surgical emergency.

Reference
Martin LW, Torres AM, *Hirschsprung's Disease*. Surg Clin North America 1985;**65**:1171–1180.

Case History 4

a)   CT brain scan (fewer marks for MRI which takes longer and is less likely to be readily available)
     Neurosurgical referral
b)   Subarachnoid haemorrhage

Key Points
- Intermittent headache or transient motor deficit can precede the haemorrhage
- Epilepsy occurs as first feature in about 20% of cases
- CT brain scan is indicated acutely, but MRI with contrast would be used to demonstrate the lesion

Reference
Aicardi J. *Disease of the Nervous System in Childhood.* Clinics in Developmental Medicine No 115/118 1992 MacKeith Press, Oxford.

Case History 5

a) Infusion of IV 10% dextrose
   Glucagon IV or IM
   Dilutional exchange transfusion
b) X-ray right arm and clavicle
   Portable doppler ultrasound of brachial and radial arteries
c) Sacral agenesis
   Hypertrophic obstructive cardiomyopathy
d) Shoulder dystocia
   Polycythaemia with thrombosis

Key Points
- Infants of diabetic mothers may become hypoglycaemic
- Macrosomia is a feature of insulin-dependent diabetic mothers
- Polycythaemia may need treatment by dilutional exchange transfusion

Discussion

Infants of insulin dependent mothers are at risk of hypoglycaemia once delivered. Neonatal hypoglycaemia is a laboratory blood glucose of less than or equal to 2.6 mmol/l. Infants with borderline low blood sugars measured by bedside tests require a sample to be sent for formal blood glucose analysis to the laboratory as the ward tests may be inaccurate for a number of reasons (e.g. polycythaemia). It may be necessary to administer IV or IM glucagon in order to elevate the blood glucose. Macrosomic infants of diabetic mothers are at risk of shoulder dystocia and subsequent Erb's palsy or fractured clavicle.

Reference
Neonatal morbidities in gestational diabetes mellitus, Diabetes Care 1998 Aug; 21 Suppl 2: B79–84 Review.

EXAM 7 : DATA INTERPRETATIONS

Question 1

a)   Blood culture, urine culture, lumbar puncture
b)   Coagulase negative staphylococcus sepsis (more marks than sepsis)
c)   Long line removal

Key Points
- Temperature instability, metabolic acidosis, high blood sugar point to sepsis

Coagulase negative staphylococcus is the commonest organism causing sepsis in preterm infants especially in association with long lines. Teicoplanin or vancomycin are the appropriate antibiotics.

Question 2

a)   Lumbar Puncture
      Cranial ultrasound scan
      EEG

Term neonatal seizures may be due to intrapartum asphyxia (first 24 hours), intracranial haemorrhage, hypoglycaemia, hypocalcaemia, congenital anomalies, drug intoxication or drug withdrawal, CNS infections, inborn errors of metabolism (first postnatal days). Infection is the commonest aetiology late in the first week and into the second week of life.

In premature infants, seizures are often due to interventricular haemorrhages. Phenobarbitone is often the first line drug of choice for control of neonatal seizures.

Question 3

a) Cortisol deficiency secondary to ACTH deficiency
   Growth hormone deficiency
   Secondary hypothyroidism
b) Hydrocortisone followed by thyroxine treatment
   GH treatment

Key Points

- GH and cortisol responses to hypoglycaemia (ITT) are flat. In an ITT if the hypoglycaemic response is adequate (decrease in blood sugar by 50% of starting value) then the GH should increase to > 13.5 mU/l to 20 and the cortisol level should increase by 100% of the basal value.
- This is a hypothalamic response to TRH. Normally in response to TRH, the TSH levels should increase at 20 mins and then decrease at 60 mins, as should the prolactin level. In this case there is an exaggerated response to TRH with the TSH levels continuing to increase at 60 mins.

Following cranial irradiation, GH insufficiency and secondary hypo-thyroidism are common. ACTH insufficiency, gonadotrophin insufficiency and diabetes insipidus are less common. Primary hypothyroidism and primary hypogonadism may also occur secondary to cranial irradiation.

Question 4

a) Schwachman-Diamond syndrome
b) Pancreatic enzyme replacements
c) Colonic fibrosis

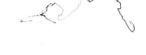

Key Points
- Pancreatic insufficiency
- Neutropenia
- Short stature
- Bony abnormalities

This syndrome of exocrine pancreatic hypoplasia, bone marrow abnormalities and metaphyseal dysplasia should be considered in the differential diagnosis of children with short stature and exocrine pancreatic disease with a normal sweat chloride. Pancreatic insufficiency may be diagnosed by measurement of stool fat output (fat balance studies) and pancreatic stimulation tests. The latter test shows that after stimulation with cholecystokinin and secretin, pancreatic enzyme output is invariably low, but in contrast to cystic fibrosis, water and bicarbonate secretion are well preserved. Faecal elastase measurement is a simpler, non-invasive test of pancreatic function as this pancreatic enzyme is not digested or absorbed by the gut and therefore low levels indicate pancreatic exocrine insufficiency.

Sepsis is usually associated with neutropenia, which may be intermittent. Thromocytopenia and hypoplastic anaemia are common.

Question 5

a) Hypernatraemic dehydration
b) 750 ml + 1000ml = 1750 ml
c) Initially normal saline

Key Points

- Hypernatraemic dehydration – proportionally more water loss than sodium
- Infants can lose fluid into bowel without obvious profuse diarrhoea
- Fluid deficit (ml) = weight (kg) x percentage dehydration x 10
- For first 10 kg of weight fluid requirement is 10 x 100 ml/day
- Aim to bring the serum sodium in hypernatraemic patient down by no more than 5 mmol/day. i.e. rehydrate over more than 48 hours
- First use normal saline, then change to e.g. 0.45% saline with 2.5% dextrose

In this condition more water is lost relative to sodium. Seizures may occur when the serum sodium is too rapidly returned to normal. During the period of dehydration, there is an increase in sodium content of cells (including brain cells). If rehydration of the relatively hypotonic fluid is too rapid, there is excessive movement of fluid into these cells.

Maintenance fluid requirements can be easily remembered by the following formula:

Body Weight	Fluid requirement per day
First 10 kg	100 ml/kg
Second 10 kg	50 ml/kg
Subsequent kg	20 ml/kg

Reference

Advanced Paediatric Life Support, 2nd edition, BMJ publishing p250

Question 6

a) Hypsarrythmia
b) Infantile spasm
c) ACTH or corticosteroids or vigabatrin

Key Points
- Chaotic pattern of high voltage arrhythmic slow waves with multifocal spikes and sharp components
- CT scan abnormal in 2/3 patients
- Developmental regression from time of seizures, occasionally before onset or seizures
- Mental retardation associated in 80–90%

Infantile spasms are generalised seizures that occur in infancy and are usually accompanied by a characteristic EEG pattern. The infantile spasms consist of sudden flexion or extension of the trunk, neck and limbs, followed by more gradual relaxation.

Question 7

a) Hereditary spherocytosis
b) Osmotic fragility test; Blood film

Key Points
- Autosomal dominant
- Unconjugated hyperbilirubinaemia
- Reticulocytosis
- Characteristic shape on blood film

HS is the most common of the hereditary haemolytic states in which there is no abnormality of the haemoglobin. The classic features are a congenital (autosomal dominant, but 25% new mutations) haemolytic process associated with splenomegaly and spherical red cells. Pigmentary gallstones usually develop in late childhood and aplastic crises associated with Parvovirus infections are the most serious complications. Lab evidence of haemolysis include reticulocytosis, anaemia and hyperbilirubinaemia. There is an abnormality in the red cell membrane, which can be demonstrated in osmotic fragility studies.

Haptoglobin binds to excess haemoglobin in the blood stream and is then excreted. A low level in this case indicates intravascular haemolysis. The treatment is splenectomy which should be deferred until the patient is 6 years of age. Polyvalent pneumococcal vaccine should be given prior to splenectomy and thereafter prophylactic penicillin is required.

Question 8

a) *Best answers – three of the following*
    Chromosomes for karyotype
    DNA testing for fragile X
    Creatinine kinase for Duchenne muscular dystrophy
    Thyroid function tests
    MRI brain scan

    Other weaker answers
    Cranial CT scan
    FBC
    Organic and amino acids

Key Points
- You are asked for useful investigations. The most useful are those that guide intervention, inform about prognosis or recurrence risk
- Duchenne muscular dystrophy often presents as developmental or speech delay. The physical findings can be subtler at a younger age.
- The fragile X phenotype become more obvious as children become older and particularly after puberty. Newer DNA tests looking for the FMR-1 mutation are both more sensitive and more specific than the original cytogenetic analysis which looked for any fragile sites.
- MRI is more sensitive to subtle abnormalities of brain development than CT. The probability of an abnormal brain scan increases with the severity of the developmental delay. Metabolic studies have a very low yield in this group of children if there are no additional clues in the history (e.g. fits/vomiting illness).

Discussion

There is little clinical consensus on appropriate investigations for this group of children. Decisions are further complicated by the high cost of investigations with low sensitivity for detecting abnormalities. The examination does not test decisions about cost-effectiveness and you should focus on the investigations which give the most useful or important information.

Question 9

a) Benign intracranial hypertension (pseudotumour cerebri)
b) CT brain
c) Monitor clinically/Acetazolamide corticosteroid treatment

Key Points
- Signs mimic those of a space occupying lesion
- Diagnostic feature of undilated ventricles in the presence of intracranial hypertension
- Sixth nerve, third and fourth nerve paresis may be seen

This condition has been described as a complication of steroid therapy (especially when the steroids are being reduced). Often the cause is obscure. The chief danger is optic nerve damage due to chronic compression. No treatment is required in many cases as there is spontaneous decrease in the raised intracranial pressure. CT scan may show a reduction in the size of the lateral ventricles because of cerebral oedema.

Question 10

a) Uncompensated respiratory acidosis due to respiratory depression (secondary to diazepam)
b) Size 5 ETT

Key Points
- ETT internal diameter (mm) = age/4 + 4. This 'easy to remember' formula is part of the APLS guidelines on resuscitation and is vital to know in an emergency.

Reference
Advanced Paediatric Life Support – 2nd edition. BMJ Publishing.

REVISION INDEX

PASTEST REVISION BOOKS

PasTest are the specialists in study guides and revision courses for professional medical qualifications. For 25 years we have been helping doctors to achieve their potential. The new PasTest range of books includes

Short Cases for the Paediatric Membership
This new book offers essential guidance for all candidates taking Paediatric Clinical examinations. The book contains summaries of popular examination cases and notes on clinical technique. Notes on approaching the Long case and Viva are also included.

R M Beattie, A T Clark & A L Smith　　　　　　**ISBN: 1 901198 25 1**

Data Interpretation for the MRCP: Revised edition
10 data interpretation practice papers with strong clinical orientation. This book provides a wide selection of data and charts reflecting the demands of the exam.

P Clark & R Neilson　　　　　　**ISBN: 1 901198 13 8**

Radiology for MRCP: 101 Cases with Discussion
This book incorporates a collection of radiological plates and discussion points for the aspiring candidate. Contains X-rays, MRI scans and CT scans with a section on understanding the principles of interpretation.

S Howling & P Jenkins　　　　　　**ISBN: 1 901198 83 5**

To order any of the above titles, please contact PasTest on Freephone

0800 980 9814

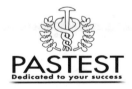

PASTEST
Dedicated to your success

PasTest, FREEPOST, Knutsford, Cheshire, WA16 7BR
Fax: 01565 650264　E-mail: books@pastest.co.uk
Web site: http://www.pastest.co.uk